Navigating Life with ADHD

David Spencer, MD, FAAN
Editor, *Brain & Life*® Books
Professor of Neurology
Oregon Health and Science University
Portland, OR

Other Titles in the *Brain & Life*® Books Series

Navigating Life with a Brain Tumor
Lynne P. Taylor, MD, FAAN; Alyx B. Porter Umphrey, MD; and Diane Richard

Navigating the Complexities of Stroke
Louis R. Caplan, MD, FAAN

Navigating Life with Epilepsy
David C. Spencer, MD, FAAN

Navigating Life with Amyotrophic Lateral Sclerosis
Mark B. Bromberg, MD, PhD, FAAN, and Diane Banks Bromberg, JD

Navigating Life with Migraine and Other Headaches
William B. Young, MD, FAAN, FANA, FAHS, and Stephen D. Silberstein, MD, FAHS, FAAN, FACP

Navigating Life with Chronic Pain
Robert A. Lavin, MD, MS; Sara Clayton, PhD; and Lindsay Zilliox, MD

Navigating Life with Parkinson's Disease, Second Edition
Sotirios A. Parashos, MD, and Rose Wichmann, PT

Navigating Life with Dementia
James M. Noble, MD, MS, CPH, FAAN

Navigating the Challenges of Concussion
Michael S. Jaffee, MD, FAAN, FANA; Donna K. Broshek, PhD, ABPP-CN; and Adrian M. Svingos, PhD

Navigating Life with Restless Legs Syndrome
Andrew R. Spector, MD, FAASM

Navigating Life with Multiple Sclerosis, Second Edition
Kathleen Costello, MS, ANP-BC, MSCN; Rosalind Kalb, PhD, CHC; and Barbara S. Giesser, MD, FAAN, FANA

Navigating Life with ADHD

Sarah Cheyette, MD
Board-Certified Pediatric Neurologist Sutter Health, San Carlos, CA

Benjamin Cheyette, MD, PhD
Board-Certified Psychiatrist, Director of ADHD Program at Mindful Health Solutions, and Professor Emeritus at the University of California, San Francisco, CA

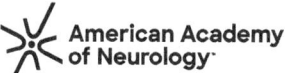
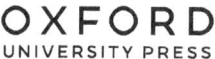

Oxford University Press is a department of the University of Oxford.
It furthers the University's objective of excellence in research, scholarship,
and education by publishing worldwide. Oxford is a registered trade mark of
Oxford University Press in the UK and certain other countries.

Published in the United States of America by Oxford University Press
198 Madison Avenue, New York, NY 10016, United States of America.

© American Academy of Neurology 2025

All rights reserved. No part of this publication may be reproduced, stored in a retrieval system, transmitted, used for text and data mining, or used for training artificial intelligence, in any form or by any means, without the prior permission in writing of Oxford University Press, or as expressly permitted by law, by license or under terms agreed with the appropriate reprographics rights organization. Inquiries concerning reproduction outside the scope of the above should be sent to the Rights Department, Oxford University Press, at the address above.

You must not circulate this work in any other form
and you must impose this same condition on any acquirer

Library of Congress Cataloging-in-Publication Data
Names: Cheyette, Sarah, 1968– author. | Cheyette, Ben, author.
Title: Navigating life with ADHD / [Sarah Cheyette, Benjamin Cheyette].
Description: New York, NY : Oxford University Press, [2025] |
Series: Brain and life books | Includes bibliographical references and index.
Identifiers: LCCN 2024041638 | ISBN 9780197646502 (paperback) |
ISBN 9780197646526 (epub) | ISBN 9780197646519 (ebook) | ISBN 9780197646533 (online)
Subjects: LCSH: Attention-deficit hyperactivity disorder—Popular works. |
Attention-deficit hyperactivity disorder—Treatment—Popular works. |
People with attention-deficit hyperactivity disorder—Popular works.
Classification: LCC RC394.A85 C44 2024 | DDC 616.85/89—dc23/eng/20241112
LC record available at https://lccn.loc.gov/2024041638

This material is not intended to be, and should not be considered, a substitute for medical or other professional advice. Treatment for the conditions described in this material is highly dependent on the individual circumstances. And, while this material is designed to offer accurate information with respect to the subject matter covered and to be current as of the time it was written, research and knowledge about medical and health issues is constantly evolving and dose schedules for medications are being revised continually, with new side effects recognized and accounted for regularly. Readers must therefore always check the product information and clinical procedures with the most up-to-date published product information and data sheets provided by the manufacturers and the most recent codes of conduct and safety regulation. The publisher and the authors make no representations or warranties to readers, express or implied, as to the accuracy or completeness of this material. Without limiting the foregoing, the publisher and the authors make no representations or warranties as to the accuracy or efficacy of the drug dosages mentioned in the material. The authors and the publisher do not accept, and expressly disclaim, any responsibility for any liability, loss or risk that may be claimed or incurred as a consequence of the use and/or application of any of the contents of this material.

DOI: 10.1093/oso/9780197646502.001.0001

Printed by Marquis Book Printing, Canada

The manufacturer's authorised representative in the EU for product safety is Oxford University Press España S.A. of El Parque Empresarial San Fernando de Henares, Avenida de Castilla, 2 - 28830 Madrid (www.oup.es/en or product.safety@ oup.com). OUP España S.A. also acts as importer into Spain of products made by the manufacturer.

CONTENTS

About the *Brain & Life*® Books Series | xiii

1. **What Is ADHD?** | 1
   What Is ADHD? | 4
   ADHD Versus ADD | 6
   The Prevalence of ADHD | 9
   ADHD in Children Versus Adults | 9
   Why Should You Do Anything About It? | 11
   The Downsides of (Untreated) ADHD | 13
       Consequences for Individuals with ADHD | 14
       Consequences on Loved Ones and Peers | 17
       Consequences on Society | 19
   The Upsides of ADHD | 19

2. **Diagnosis: Where and How to Get Help** | 23
   Who Is the Right Professional to Diagnose My ADHD? | 23
   Should You See a Psychologist (PhD) or a Physician (MD)? | 24
   What Will Your Initial Doctor's Visit for ADHD Be Like? | 26
   A Brief History of ADHD Diagnosis | 29
   What You Can Learn from the History of ADHD | 31

Current Diagnostic Criteria for ADHD | 32
   Inattention-Related Symptoms | 32
   Symptoms Related to Hyperactivity and Impulsivity | 33
Tests That Help Diagnose ADHD | 38
Do I (or Does My Child) Need Neuropsychological Testing for ADHD? | 42
Should I (or My Child) Get a Genetic Test or Brain Scan for ADHD? | 46
   Genetic Testing | 46
   Brain Scans | 47

3. **What Causes ADHD? Biology** | 49
   A Permission Slip for Our Readers | 49
   Are Any Brain Structures Abnormal or Different in ADHD? | 50
   Differences in Brain Growth in ADHD | 53
   Diagnostic Implications of Brain Anatomy and Brain Growth Studies | 53
   What About Differences in Brain Function? | 54
   What Brain Chemicals Are Involved in ADHD? | 55
   Hope for the Future: Combining Brain Anatomy with Brain Chemistry | 60
   The Role of Heredity (Genes) in ADHD | 60
   Is ADHD Partly a Matter of Chance? | 62
   Summary: Implications of Biology for ADHD Diagnosis and Treatment | 63

4. **What Causes ADHD? Society and Environment** | 65
   Contributions of the Environment and Culture to ADHD | 65
      Drug Use | 67
         Prenatal Drug Exposure | 67
         Postnatal Drug Use | 67

Psychological Stress | 68
    Prenatal Exposure | 68
    Stress During Infancy | 69
    During Childhood and Adolescence | 69
Toxins | 70
Sugar, Artificial Ingredients, and Artificial Colors | 70
Dietary Supplements | 71
Electronic Distractions/Diversions | 72
"Crazy Busy" Lives | 75

ADHD in Marginalized Communities | 79

Contributions from Other Mental Health Challenges | 80

5. **Could My ADHD Actually Be Something Else?** | 83

How Other Factors Can Mimic or Worsen ADHD | 83

Psychiatric Conditions | 84
    Depression | 89
    Anxiety | 90
        How Anxiety and Depression Can Mimic ADHD | 90
    Bipolar Disorder | 92
    Obsessive–Compulsive Disorder (OCD) | 92
    Psychosis | 93

Autism Spectrum Disorder (ASD) | 94

Dementia | 96

Addiction | 98

Poor Sleep | 98

Medical Conditions | 101
    Obstructive Sleep Apnea | 101
    Absence Seizures | 102
    Conditions that Cause Fatigue or Pain | 103

6. **Treatment with Medications** | 104

   What Makes It So Hard to Decide Whether to Take a
      Medication? | 104

   Addressing Parental Fears | 108

   What Can I, My Partner, or My Child Hope to Get out of Taking
      a Medication? | 109

   The Decision to Take Medication | 110

   Choosing a Medication | 112

   Genetic Testing to Optimize Medication Choice | 113

   What Kinds of ADHD Medication Are There? | 115

   Side Effects of Stimulant Medications | 118
   - Insomnia | 118
   - Weight Loss | 118
   - Mood Changes and Irritability | 119
   - Increased Heart Rate and Blood Pressure | 119
   - Addiction | 120
   - Miscellaneous | 121

   Types of Stimulants | 121
   - Methylphenidate-Based Stimulant Medications
       (Ritalin) | 122
   - Amphetamine-Based Stimulant Medications
       (Adderall) | 125

   Brand-Name Versus Generic Medication | 126

   Nonstimulants | 128

   Off-Label Medications | 130

   What about Caffeine? | 131

   Dosing | 132

   How Often Will I Need to See My Doctor? | 133

   Supplements | 133

   Limitations of Medication-Based Treatments in Psychiatric
      Conditions | 134

7. **Coaching and Therapy Tips | 136**

   Talk-Based Treatment Approaches: Coaching Versus Therapy | 137

   Types of Talk Therapy | 139

   Some Useful Coaching and Therapy Tips | 142
   Set Goals | 142
   Celebrate Each Success | 143
   Visualization | 145
   Improve Time Management | 145
   Interval Training | 146
   Identify Your Own Lies | 147
   Keep a To-Do List and Set Reminders | 147
   Practice Mindfulness | 148
   Remove Your "Self" from the Situation | 148
   Practice Situation Selection Awareness | 148
   Improve Communication Skills | 150
   Couples Therapy | 151
   Organization Therapy | 151
   Rest and Relax | 152
   Get Sufficient Exercise | 152
   Get Enough Sleep | 153

8. **Procrastination: A Major Problem for Most People with ADHD | 154**

   Procrastination | 154

   Identifying Ambivalence | 156

   Understanding the ADHDer's Viewpoint | 157

   Skills to Manage Procrastination | 159
   Get Help with Your Personal Blocks | 159
   Start with the Smallest Bit | 159
   Break Large, Complex Tasks Down into Smaller, Achievable Chunks | 160
   Schedule Dreaded Tasks Early | 160

Recognize and End "Procrastivity" | 162
Impose Negative Consequences for Inaction | 162
Manage Electronic Distractions | 164

9. **Help in School and Self-Directed Treatments** | 166

Help in School: 504 Plans, Individualized Education Programs, and Other Accommodations | 166

Are Accommodations a Good Idea? | 168

Accommodations at Work | 170

Self-Help: Blogs, Vlogs, Books, Support Groups, and Other Resources | 170

Electronic Aids (Apps, Websites, and Other Tools) | 171

Technology-Based Treatments for ADHD | 171

10. **ADHD Across the Lifespan** | 174

How ADHD Is Different in Children Versus Adults | 174
  Biological Factors, Part 1: The Developing Brain | 175
  Biological Factors, Part 2: Sex and Gender | 178
  Psychosocial Factors, Part 1: School and Work | 180
    Preschool | 181
    Elementary School | 182
    Middle School | 183
    High School | 184
    College | 187
    Adulthood | 188
  Special Issues When ADHD Adults Become Parents | 191
    ADHD in Pregnant and Breastfeeding Moms | 192
  Psychosocial Factors, Part 2: ADHD in the Family | 193

Differences in Therapeutic Approaches in Children Versus Adults | 196

Incorporating Differences in ADHD Across the Lifespan into Diagnostic Criteria | 201

11. **For Care Partners** | 203

   What Does It Mean to Be a Care Partner? | 203

   Acknowledging Feelings and Fears | 205
   - Anger | 205
   - Fear | 205
   - Shame | 206
   - Guilt | 206

   Getting Help | 209

   Focus on the Positives | 211

   Understand the Invisible Symptoms of ADHD | 212

   When to Support Versus When to Step Back | 214

   Find Ways to Connect to the ADHDer in Your Life | 217

   Make Time for Yourself | 218

   Summary | 218

12. **The Gift of ADHD** | 219

GLOSSARY | 223
APPENDIX 1: FURTHER RESOURCES | 243
APPENDIX 2: HII-5 | 251
ABOUT *BRAIN & LIFE*® AND THE AMERICAN ACADEMY OF NEUROLOGY | 253
INDEX | 255

ABOUT THE *BRAIN & LIFE*® BOOKS SERIES

What was the first thing you thought when you learned you or a family member had a neurologic disease? Perhaps you were confused, uncertain, afraid, or maybe even in denial. A common thread is often the realization that life has changed and may continue to change, but also uncertainty about exactly what that means or what to expect. And yet, neurologic diseases themselves inevitably change—sometimes quickly, in a matter of seconds or minutes, and sometimes gradually over months or even years.

With any new diagnosis—especially one that is potentially life-changing—you may not be prepared to take in and process large amounts of new information on the spot. And even under the best circumstances, each condition comes with the need to learn a new language and understand the necessary tests, underlying causes, and right treatments. It may be difficult to wrap your arms around a great deal of information in what are often time-limited appointments with your neurologist. Understanding your new diagnosis and how to manage it is a gradual process, and you will inevitably have questions with the passage of time and reflection. Learning about your condition can help you understand what the most useful and accurate information is to share with your neurology team, allowing you to fully participate in treatment decisions.

But facts and information are only part of the picture. You may have questions about how to manage your day-to-day life with a neurologic disease, whether in terms of your career, your home, your relationships, or, in some instances, long-term planning and care. We designed the *Brain & Life* Books series to help you address some of the fears, concerns, and difficult emotions you may feel, such as grief and worry, by harnessing the power of accurate and timely information to help guide you and your family through the changes brought about by a neurologic diagnosis. The books share stories of others who have traveled down paths like the one you are on to reinforce the fact that you are not alone.

We selected the authors of the series carefully with these goals in mind. First and foremost, all authors are respected experts in their field, and the information in the *Brain & Life* Books series is accurate, up-to-date, and written to be understandable to someone with no medical background. Experts from the leading professional neurology organization in the world—the American Academy of Neurology—and the oldest and largest university press in the world—Oxford University Press—carefully review each book to ensure the highest quality. But we also chose our authors because of their experience and ability to connect with patients and their families. The experiences and feelings you are having now have been dealt with and managed successfully by our authors and their patients. Our authors will share with you best practices, stories, and pearls of advice that will leave you with a feeling that your diagnosis is manageable—you can do this. We have highlighted all key terms that you and your family should know when first used, and we have included them in a comprehensive glossary at the back of the book.

The *Brain & Life* Books series was written with you in mind, whether you have been diagnosed yourself or are a family member, caregiver, or friend of someone who has been, as a resource for successfully navigating life with a neurologic disease.

David Spencer, MD, FAAN
Editor, *Brain & Life*® Books
Professor of Neurology
Oregon Health and Science University,
Portland, OR

CHAPTER 1

What Is ADHD?

In this chapter, you will learn:

- What ADHD is
- How common ADHD is in children versus adults
- Why you should do anything about it
- The downsides of (untreated) ADHD
- The upsides of ADHD

So—you want to learn about **attention-deficit/hyperactivity disorder (ADHD)**.

You may be reading this book because a teacher or school administrator shared concerns about how your child is doing in class. The school also said your child should see some kind of specialist—but which kind? Maybe this has got you thinking about yourself and whether you have ADHD too. After all, everybody says you and your kid are alike—and not just in looks, but also in the way you speak and behave. Or perhaps your **therapist** mentioned you might have ADHD. You started therapy because you felt depressed or anxious and your doctor recommended it. You weren't looking for help with attention, but after a few sessions, your therapist said you should look into getting tested for ADHD. They also said they can't make an ADHD diagnosis themselves. Why not? Who are you supposed to see for a diagnosis now that this issue has been raised? Or maybe you've come to suspect you have ADHD on your own after hearing about it on a podcast or seeing a video on TikTok or YouTube. You looked at your phone and thought: "Hey, that's just like me!" So now what?

There's a lot of oversimplified information—or, worse, misinformation—out there about ADHD: on the internet, from friends and acquaintances, even sometimes from therapists or in books. ADHD is a complicated subject: It involves **biology, psychology**, and medicine, as well as cultural expectations about how kids and adults are supposed to behave and perform. We intend this book to provide accurate, up-to-date information about ADHD: what it is, how to diagnose it, how to treat it, how to live with it, and what to expect from it throughout a lifetime—whether that is your own lifetime or that of your child.

> *Pete is 42. He admits he was "somewhat of a troublemaker" in grade school but got "OK" grades, mainly Bs and Cs, often relying on charm to wrangle deadline extensions out of his teachers. He felt he was "never really smart" and also a bit "lazy" (his parents' words, which later became his own) but he has always taken pride in being a "people person." He went to college and had a great time—barely scraping by academically. But he had no problems finding a job in sales after graduation, in part because of the many contacts he had made in his fraternity. Thereafter, although he was excellent at the sales part of his job, he was not promoted by his first employer and was fired by his second due to missed deadlines and sloppy paperwork. He comes in for a psychological evaluation because of a "nagging feeling that I could have been better." He is also now father to a son who he notes is charting a similar course in school so far. He wants to guide his son better than his parents guided him.*

ADHD affects many, many people—including those who don't have it! If you don't have ADHD yourself and have picked up this book because you are the parent, spouse, or caregiver of someone with ADHD, then you already know exactly what we mean: ADHD alters your life when it affects someone you love, especially if they are someone you live with. But even if you don't have a family member or partner with ADHD, it is such a common condition that it likely still impacts your life.

If you're the parent of a child with ADHD, you may frequently find yourself in the position of either having to defend or discipline your child. You may struggle with how much of your child's behavior to excuse versus how much to punish; how much is the right amount of support for your child versus too much; when is it necessary to rein them in and when is it OK to just let your kid be a kid. You may have found you must constantly come up with creative parenting solutions because the "usual methods" that work for other children don't work for your child. The impulsiveness of an ADHD child can create serious family distress. And as the child ages into adolescence, this often goes beyond academic and disciplinary struggles in school; it can include things like drug use and a higher rate of traumatic accidents due to impulsive risk-taking behaviors.

If you're the significant other of an adult with ADHD, you may be grappling with a partner who doesn't listen or attend to what you say—even when you think it is important. You may be frustrated with a partner who at times acts in ways that seem extremely irresponsible. This may be even more frustrating if that same partner seems to act responsibly at work and yet is lackadaisical with your shared or family chores. It can be hard not to take that personally.

If you're the adult child of an older parent with ADHD, you may be able to keep track of things and wonder why your mother or father never did when you were growing up. You may feel you had to "grow up too quickly" and take on responsibilities for them when it should have been the reverse: They should have been the ones taking on responsibility for you. Maybe they were less present or even absent from your life—for reasons arising at least in part from their struggles with ADHD—including broken relationships, criminal behavior, or substance abuse. You may fear that their behavior has transgenerational consequences; that is, that your ongoing issues with your parent could adversely affect the way you parent your own children.

That is not to mention others with ADHD whom you routinely interact with outside your family, such as teachers, students, employers, bosses, direct reports, coworkers, friends, strangers—even just other drivers on the road! ADHD is such a common condition that everyone interacts with people with this condition. The fact is that ADHD has consequences for everybody in society.

What Is ADHD?

ADHD is classified by most experts as a **neurodevelopmental** disorder; that is, that it results from differences in the way the brain develops. Whereas ADHD was once thought to be a disorder exclusively affecting school-aged children, it is now clear that most children with ADHD grow up to be adults with ADHD. The common symptoms of ADHD are full of opposites. They include inattention as well as occasionally paying too much attention to the wrong things or to one thing in particular. They include the tendency to sit and daydream as well as the tendency to be hyperactive and behaviorally disruptive in certain settings. Some people who don't have ADHD think they do or believe they benefit from the medications used to treat it, but even more people probably have it without realizing or seeking treatment for it. Since ADHD can masquerade as many other conditions, including **depression** and **anxiety**, doctors and other medical professionals often miss it or mistake it for something else. Even so, there is a pervasive fear that it is overdiagnosed and that medications used to treat it are overprescribed or abused. ADHD is dismissed as a joke by some and considered a serious disability by others. It is a consequence of the way your brain is wired—that is, your innate mental strengths and weaknesses—but also of your habits, your environment, and the demands placed upon you.

Alanna always got good grades. What grade-school teachers (and her parents) didn't fully appreciate was that she frequently procrastinated until the last second and pulled "all-nighters" to complete assignments on time, or was so distracted that she spent hours on assignments that should have taken only 30 minutes. Internally, she felt like an imposter, a fraud: She didn't deserve all the compliments she received about her school performance because the people who made them didn't realize how long it took her to do even simple assignments, or that she typically did everything at the last minute.

Alanna went to college, where—with the increased academic workload—her problems increased. She hardly slept and pulled more and more all-nighters to meet deadlines. She was so fearful of disappointing her family that she pushed herself beyond reasonable limits until she finally experienced a "nervous breakdown" and attempted suicide.

*The first **psychiatrist** who saw her after her breakdown treated her for depression, but she did not benefit from trials of several different **antidepressants**. She continued to have low self-esteem and to struggle academically and personally. Nobody, including the psychiatrist, thought to ask her questions about her longstanding issues with attention regulation. Only much later, when a different psychiatrist finally diagnosed Alanna with ADHD and treated her for it, did her depression permanently lift. It was at this point in her life, in her 30s, that she finally started to gain a new self-image: realizing that she was not, and never had been, a fraud. She was actually a very smart and ambitious person with defined and treatable attention issues. She often said, "My life began again at age 30, with my ADHD diagnosis."*

ADHD Versus ADD

When we first start explaining to a new patient about ADHD, some respond with: "I don't have ADHD, I have **ADD**." By this, they mean they have only inattentive symptoms—they have never had issues with hyperactivity or controlling their behavior in school or at work. Attention-deficit disorder (ADD) is an older name for the condition that is now considered a subtype of ADHD according to the most recent *Diagnostic and Statistical Manual of Psychiatric Disorders* (DSM-5); that is, there is no separate condition called "ADD." Some people with ADHD only have symptoms of hyperactivity and impulsivity; others only have symptoms of inattentiveness but aren't hyperactive or impulsive; and some have both sets of symptoms. All are diagnosed with the same **neuropsychiatric** condition: ADHD (though their specific **presentation** may be further specified as "predominantly inattentive," "predominantly hyperactive," or "combined"). There are some good reasons for this convention, which we will describe in later chapters (for instance, "The Role of Heredity" in Chapter 3). For now, suffice it to say that throughout this book we follow the official current naming convention: When we say "ADHD," we mean all of the conditions described above, including what used to be called "ADD."

Already you can see that answering the question "What is ADHD?" isn't so simple, but here is a simple way to think about it:

> Everybody focuses sometimes. "Focusing" means paying attention to one input from the environment while setting aside all other inputs as less important. It's like having one important paper out on your desk while everything else is put away in drawers. Your brain sees only the one thing it needs to see and, as a result, it can spend uninterrupted time on it, do it well, and complete it in the right amount of time. And that feels great! People who focus well feel great about what

they accomplish, and that typically translates into feeling great about themselves. In other words, with focus comes confidence and self-esteem. Confidence means feeling hopeful and optimistic about your ability to tackle new challenges in the future. A person who can focus is able to get things done and, with repetition, grows to believe in their abilities and to see themselves as a success story. This is a **virtuous cycle**: If you believe you are a successful person who is good at getting things done, you will continue to work hard to get things done. When you are faced with a new challenge, you will put in the effort required to find a solution and keep going. You will do this in no small part because you have internalized a view of yourself as a successful person—and successful people find solutions and work hard to overcome challenges.

Everybody is also unfocused sometimes. In an unfocused state, many inputs from the environment feel equally important, and so you are more likely to transition or "flit" from one input to another. In contrast to our earlier example, when you're not focused you no longer have a single piece of paper on your desk with all the others tucked away in drawers. Instead, you have many pieces of paper out on your desk that all compete for your attention. In this state, your brain "sees" a lot of different disconnected things—not really all at once, but in a rapid succession that may feel simultaneous at times. This can have advantages—it can lead to novel ideas, as your brain knits disparate concepts together, connecting ideas that were previously unrelated. But from a productivity standpoint, although your brain is active in this state, it may have trouble completing any single multi-step or complex task because it keeps getting diverted from one task or thought to another. It's important to note that this state of mind is not in itself abnormal or **pathological**. Everybody spends some time in this mental state—it is often experienced as daydreaming, but it may also be linked to creativity, artistic expression, and even some

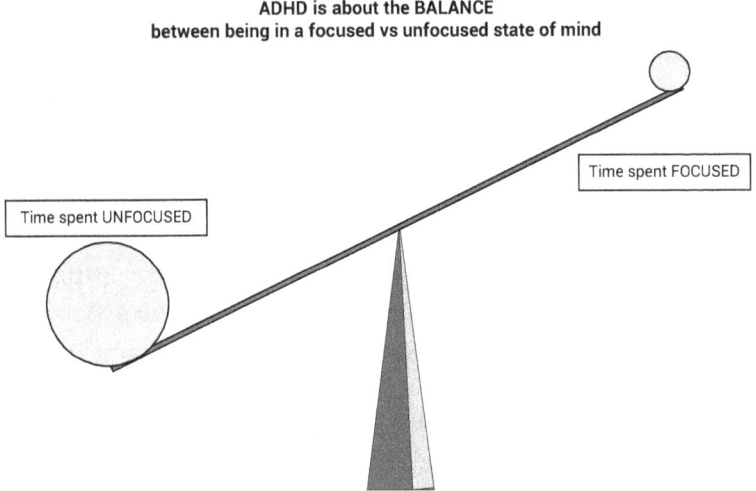

FIGURE 1.1 Having ADHD does not mean you can't focus at all. Instead, it means you have difficulties regulating your attention, and as a result spend too much time in an "unfocused" state or too much time focusing on one thing in particular.

aspects of athletic performance. It is sometimes known as being "in the flow."

If everybody is focused sometimes and unfocused sometimes, what does it mean to have ADHD? Simply put, ADHD means you spend too much time in an unfocused state (Figure 1.1). This might mean you almost never focus well, but it could also mean you have difficulty transitioning into or maintaining a focused state when called upon to do so. In day-to-day terms, this means you have challenges getting some types of tasks done and/or behaving as required in certain situations—for example, in class or at work meetings. A person with ADHD will often have difficulty sitting still or controlling their impulses in situations where consideration of others is required. They will procrastinate and not complete tasks on time or at all, and when they do complete tasks, they will often feel the outcome doesn't represent their true ability.

The Prevalence of ADHD

According to the most recent government and clinical survey data, the **prevalence** of ADHD in the United States is about 9% to 10% in children and about 4% to 5% in adults. For comparison, the prevalence of **major depressive episode** in adults in the United States is about 8.5%, and the prevalence of **generalized anxiety disorder** is about 3%. Thus, in terms of how common it is, ADHD is among the top three major psychiatric conditions (excluding all forms of substance abuse) in the adult population of the United States.

There are a few important points to make about these numbers for ADHD. In general, ADHD is more commonly diagnosed in males than in females; this may be due to gender biases regarding cultural and societal expectations as well as to some biological differences between the sexes. Also, although ADHD is currently about twice as common among children compared to adults, it was only recently, with the publication of DSM-5 in 2013, that criteria for adult ADHD were established by the American Psychiatric Association; ever since that change, diagnosis rates in adults have been climbing rapidly. Logically, even allowing that some children do eventually "grow out of it," since ADHD is now thought to be a lifelong condition for most people, the prevalence rates in children and adults should be more similar. In fact, we expect diagnosis rates in adults to continue to climb and that rates in children and adults will converge as the recognition and understanding of ADHD grows and stabilizes among professionals who treat adults.

ADHD in Children Versus Adults

In our many years of treating patients with ADHD, we have experienced innumerable occasions when a child came in for diagnosis/treatment and, over the course of our evaluation, one or both of their parents had an epiphany: "Hey, I have ADHD, too!" In some cases, the struggles of the parent had never before been brought to light; it was only in talking about the struggles of their child that the parent suddenly realized, "That's me, too!" In other cases, the parent could recall concerns that had been raised about their own behavior when they were a child (often by a teacher) but had been set aside by their parents and never accepted or addressed, most often because of stigma or cultural resistance to the concept of mental illness or its treatment.

As we will discuss in Chapters 2 and 4, although ADHD has probably been around for as long as humans, the diagnosis of what we now call ADHD only emerged in the last century. It initially stemmed from concerns about the ability of some school-aged children to pay attention, sit still, remain quiet, and follow instructions in traditional classroom settings. As mentioned in the paragraph above about prevalence rates, only in the last few decades has the medical community come to recognize and embrace that, for many if not most of the people who have it, ADHD continues to create challenges into adulthood.

As physicians, we take this extremely seriously. Simply put, for most people who have it, ADHD is a lifelong condition with significant consequences at all ages. Unlike many books about ADHD that focus on either children or adults, in this book we are addressing ADHD at all ages. There are some differences in the presentation and challenges of ADHD at different stages of life that we will discuss in Chapter 10. But for now, suffice it to say that from a medical perspective, childhood ADHD and adult ADHD are far more alike than different. The primary symptoms are identical, whether one is talking about **inattentiveness, hyperactivity, impulsivity**, or (as is increasingly being recognized) **affective reactivity/lability**. Treatment is also identical or very similar: With few exceptions, both the medications and mental coping and behavioral strategies for ADHD are the same for children and adults. And while there are some emerging technologies for ADHD diagnosis or treatment that have so far only been approved by the U.S. Food and Drug

Administration (FDA) in children, that is likely only temporary. There is little reason to believe that a device or app that can diagnose, treat, or help manage ADHD in children and teens won't work for ADHD in adults.

Why Should You Do Anything About It?

Even if we don't yet completely understand it, there is ample evidence that ADHD has a biological basis (discussed more fully in Chapter 3); it is a legitimate medical diagnosis. Still, compared to other medical concerns, many people mistakenly feel the negative impacts of untreated ADHD are not as clear or consequential as for some other medical conditions. ADHD might not seem as likely to hurt or kill you, but there are significant negative consequences to not treating ADHD both in children and adults. These include serious consequences on health and even on mortality.

> *Zachary achieved occasional high marks throughout his school years, especially on projects he found interesting. He was always popular, was pretty good at sports, and had plenty of friends, but as academics got more challenging in high school and college, he ran into increasing trouble completing assignments on time. He got a pass from his teachers in high school, but in college he was forced to repeat two required courses due to incomplete assignments. That's not even counting a few other courses that he only passed because of sympathetic professors who granted him deadline extensions. Still, he managed to graduate along with the rest of his classmates—even if it was just by the skin of his teeth.*
>
> *After college, Zachary struggled to hold down a job. He constantly fell behind on his workload. He couldn't get motivated to start or finish the more mundane tasks required of his*

work, even after being reprimanded repeatedly by supervisors. This eventually led to termination and a search for a new job. He did well on job interviews, and each new position started out OK, but in a matter of months, he would find himself in hot water again over his backlog of incomplete work. With each repeated cycle of this pattern, Zachary became increasingly convinced that each time he was hired, it was only a matter of time before he'd get fired and have to look for a new job again. As a result he started to make less and less of an effort to avoid the outcome he already viewed as inevitable. That was OK until, eventually, all his personal charm could not overcome his patchy résumé and work history—and he stopped getting hired altogether.

Zachary's inability to organize and complete tasks also had other damaging effects on his life. Several intimate relationships failed due to the frustrations of his partners over his unreliability, apparent inattention, and occasionally impulsive behavior, not to mention his inability to hold down a steady job and get promoted. After his last serious girlfriend gave up on him, he lost the confidence to try for another relationship. He stopped dating and actively avoided any potentially serious partners who crossed his path.

He eventually found himself living in his parents' house. His friends from high school and college had all moved on with their lives—they were stably employed, and most were married and had started having children. He stopped exercising or playing sports, gained a lot of weight, and spent most of his time playing videogames, drinking beer, and smoking cannabis on the couch in his parents' basement.

Although it shocked him the first time it crossed his mind, it eventually became habitual: He just couldn't shake the nagging thought that his life wasn't worth living.

The Downsides of (Untreated) ADHD

The question of "What are the consequences of untreated ADHD?" or, to put it another way, "Why should we diagnose or treat this condition?" is no less important than "What is ADHD?" Most people are aware that school-aged children and college students with ADHD may benefit from treatment to help them get through classes without being distracted or too disruptive to their peers and to enable them to get their assignments done and sit through tests. But what about after schooling is over? Why does it matter if adults who are done with school never get treated for ADHD?

The consequences of untreated (or undertreated) ADHD in adults can be severe: This is true for individuals with the disorder, for the people close to them, and for society as a whole. Untreated ADHD is a serious medical condition linked to:

- Increased risk of accidents, including motor vehicle accidents and brain injuries
- Increased exposure to violence, both as a perpetrator and as a victim
- Increased early childbearing
- Increased promiscuity and exposure to sexually transmitted diseases
- Increased chaotic household environment
- Increased divorce rate
- Increased legal problems, bankruptcy, and criminal activity
- Increased risk of depression, anxiety, and suicide
- Increased risk of substance abuse and substance dependence
- Increased risk of medical problems linked to poor impulse control (for example, poor diet and lack of exercise), such as **diabetes**, **heart disease**, and stroke
- Lower overall life expectancy due to all of the above.

Consequences for Individuals with ADHD

When you grow up feeling like you never finish tasks, frequently do things wrong, and make a lot of errors or mistakes, who do you tend to become? There is the easy answer that failing to accomplish tasks in school leads to not going far in your education, and this then impacts your career opportunities and choices thereafter. While there are many, many stories of successful people who do not have a college degree, most of us would agree that completing your education and doing it well has advantages when it comes to your subsequent ability to make a living and support yourself and a family.

But treating ADHD is not just about getting good grades, completing a degree, and using that to get a good job or start a career. In school, if you have untreated ADHD you may not turn in homework or fail a class, and there will be consequences from parents and teachers. They may get angry with you, and your grades will go down. That may seem like a big deal (and it is), but just compare it to what can happen to adults with untreated ADHD: If you have trouble fulfilling the duties of your job due to ADHD symptoms, consequences may include not getting promoted or even getting fired. And it's worth noting that the consequences of ADHD, including those occurring in a work setting, can get worse as you get older. Far from "outgrowing" and leaving behind childhood ADHD symptoms (as used to be the widespread clinical view), there is evidence that many adults with ADHD encounter new difficulties as they age. This is because tasks and responsibilities get more difficult and complex in adulthood, and also because social and work expectations are often more restrictive for fully mature adults than for children or college-age young adults. This is often evident in people with ADHD who are otherwise academically gifted and so manage to get good grades or go to college or graduate school despite significant attentional challenges. Until recently, it was thought that if you did well enough in school to get a professional degree, you couldn't possibly have ADHD.

> Jayson was quick-witted, social, and knowledgeable in a wide range of subjects and could remember things easily once he learned them. Because of this he could be a lot of fun at large gatherings. In college, he was popular among his peers but also had a reputation among friends and acquaintances for never getting started on projects until the last minute and for pulling "all-nighter marathons" to finish his work. That said, although he was often bleary-eyed and "crashed" in bed for a whole day after a deadline, what he produced was typically of excellent quality, and he managed to graduate from a top university with a degree in computer engineering.
>
> He initially did well in his post-college work life as an engineer. As in college, he got all his work done just at deadline, but since it was always of high quality and often exceeded expectations, he was rapidly promoted within his company.
>
> As a result of promotion, he was increasingly required to sit in on planning and managerial meetings, to which he was often late. He frequently did not seem to be listening, was easily distracted by his computer and phone, and did not speak for long stretches. When he did open his mouth, it was often to interrupt others—and what he said revealed he was either stuck on a topic that the group had already moved on from, or that his mind had raced ahead (or sideways) compared to everyone else in the room.

Beyond its effects on your ability to complete tasks efficiently, untreated ADHD also can affect your emotional health and self-perception. People with ADHD often experience increasingly negative interactions with other people as they mature. They begin to hear the following phrases *a lot*:

- "Whaddya mean you forgot?!"
- "You didn't listen."

- "You should have done better."
- "What's wrong with you? Why can't you just __?"

This negative feedback adds up over time. It's been said that to develop a good self-image, a child needs to hear three or four encouragements for every criticism. Well, kids with ADHD often hear 30 criticisms for every encouragement. As a result, many kids with ADHD, as they are developing an idea of their own self-worth, wind up feeling very negative about themselves. The people they most love and respect (parents, teachers, coaches) use words like "lazy," "irresponsible," or just plain "bad" to describe them. These kids often develop into adults with poor self-esteem.

This creates a **vicious cycle**: A person with ADHD fails often, hears lots of criticism, and grows to doubt their abilities—they are therefore more likely to fail. Often people with ADHD—both kids and adults—know they are intelligent yet struggle with a very poor self-image. They feel they should be able to do things but don't feel confident that they will be able to. Or they just don't know what's wrong with them: "I don't understand why it's so much easier for everyone else." They have learned to say and think to themselves: "I'm no good at spreadsheets" or "School is not for me." They often give up on tasks before they even begin: "Why bother? I'm just going to make a mistake." Of course these thoughts are both self-defeating and self-reinforcing because they make you even less likely to focus on trying to succeed in these types of activities. And when something does go wrong, instead of making an effort to find solutions, you are more likely to give up.

> *Andrea always got good grades in middle school, but unlike most of her friends who took about an hour to complete their homework, she often took 3. She wanted to do well, so she did whatever it took, but as a result, she had no time to develop other interests or hobbies. Her middle-school teachers did not realize*

> this about her; neither did her parents. Her teachers saw completed work, and her parents saw A's on a report card—nobody realized that these results came at a personal cost different from that of her peers.
>
> Now that Andrea is 14 and in high school, things have taken a turn for the worse: Her 3 hours of nightly homework have ballooned into more than 6. Her grades are suffering, and yet because of all the time she spends struggling to keep up academically, she has no time for other outlets that might buttress her happiness or contribute to her self-esteem. She has become more socially isolated and depressed. Her motivation is deteriorating because she has begun to feel she can't succeed. "What's the use?" she thinks. "Everyone else is smarter than me. I'll never get into a good college. And why should I bother even trying? Even if I do get in, that will be even harder. I'll never be able to survive."

This negative self-talk has significant consequences as you get older, consequences that get to the heart of how you feel about your capabilities and about yourself as a human being. Do you view yourself as someone who does what they set out to do? As someone who has realized their potential? Do you feel respected by others, and do you respect yourself? Or do you feel like a failure who has repeatedly let yourself and others down? Can you be trusted with responsibility? Should you be promoted or volunteer to take on something important? Or would you and everybody else be better off if you just did your best to stay where you are and fade into the background?

Consequences on Loved Ones and Peers

ADHD impacts relationships with others as well as your relationship with yourself. The feedback "You never listen!" does not enhance romance, partnership, or bonding. Forgetfulness in a personal relationship is often interpreted as "You don't care." If you say you're going to do the dishes but don't, your partner will see you as irresponsible and untrustworthy. They may get impatient with repeated promises that never pan out, or with ventures that repeatedly fail for the same reasons—reasons they may find hard to understand the cause of, such as never finishing what you begin or always missing deadlines.

> *Jim's wife, Eva, is furious with him. He promised to take their son Michael to baseball practice this Saturday morning after he finished his workout, but didn't show up in time and didn't respond to her texts to see where he was. She had plans to take a break and get her hair done, but canceled at the last minute and bundled Michael into the car to take him to practice herself.*
>
> *When Jim finally shows up 40 minutes late to the practice, he initially acts as though nothing is amiss, chatting loudly with the other dads and calling out fatherly advice to Michael. Eventually he approaches Eva, and an embarrassing argument rapidly ensues. It turns out Eva is angry not just about this one incident. She recites a litany of Jim's failures as both a father and a spouse: She can't rely on him, he never listens to her, he is always forgetting appointments, he promises to get things done around the house but somehow never accomplishes anything on his "to-do list," he forgets about his son's practices and games, and he doesn't even help him with his homework. Eva works for a living too (thanks to a recent promotion, she actually makes more than Jim), yet she is also the one who pulls off everything at home, including picking up all the slack that Jim never gets done. Eva would simply like him to contribute something—anything!—to help her out a little bit.*
>
> *He apologizes profusely and promises it won't happen again, but she tells him to save his breath. As she picks up her things to go, she advises him that he'd be better off spending some time finding a good divorce attorney.*

Consequences on Society

ADHD has societal consequences, too. For starters, ADHD essentially robs directly from the economy by reducing worker productivity. But beyond this, ADHD also robs society of the potential creative and other contributions that individuals with ADHD might be able to make if their symptoms were well controlled. In other words, there are great ideas that never come to fruition. Additionally, untreated ADHD can also be dangerous, both for the individuals who have it and for the bystanders around them. People with ADHD tend to be risk-takers and are more impulsive. When they are younger, this may translate into increased participation in activities where they might get broken bones or a concussion. They often engage in situations where they "test gravity," such as jumping off the tops of objects that should never even be climbed on. The consequences of these tendencies become more dire, especially for others, as the person with ADHD ages into adulthood. To take just one common example, having uncontrolled ADHD while driving (especially when combined with being distracted by a phone in the car) can be fatal—both for the driver and for their passengers, and for people in the cars they collide with and those who are just in the wrong place at the wrong time.

Untreated ADHD also contributes to drinking and illicit drug use, both as an impulsive thrill-seeking behavior and also to escape what is often the painful reality of unfulfilled potential. With drug use can come further dangerous behaviors such as reckless driving, unprotected sex, domestic violence, and criminal activity. Unrecognized and untreated ADHD is often a linchpin in a vicious cycle of negative behavior that leads to increasingly poor outcomes for the individual with ADHD as well as those around them.

The Upsides of ADHD

"But wait," the ADHDer might say. "If you never take chances, the world does not move forward. Without some impulsivity, nobody would start a business. Nobody would do anything different. Life's not just about playing it safe and getting work done. It's about thinking of new things to do! It's about being creative, putting things together in a different way! The world owes us ADHDers a debt of gratitude!" We agree.

Some people with ADHD consider it their "superpower." For some, it means less dithering around, less fear of pursuing novel ideas—no matter how "out of the box" those ideas may be. People with ADHD often thrive in jobs that are physically active, require switching gears frequently to creatively solve new problems, and/or require a lot of "putting out fires"—whether figuratively (in an office setting) or literally (such as working as an emergency responder).

Sometimes ADHD is an asset socially. An ADHDer's energy can come across as very charismatic, and they may develop a reputation for being super-fun to be around. They may be more likely to try new experiences and thereby gain a lot of personal growth. While their peers were plodding through college or graduate school, they might have been trekking across a continent off the beaten track and experiencing adventures few people ever have.

Physically, relatively lax impulse control can be a benefit in sports or athletic endeavors. The same little kid whose energy leads them to defy gravity by jumping off the top of the swing set may use that same tendency to take risks in skiing that ultimately lead them to become an Olympic-level freestyle champion. The ability to notice a lot of details at once can also be helpful in sports. For example, a basketball player needs to be able to focus not just on the ball, but also on where their opponents are, where their teammates are, and the signals their teammates are using to show that they are open.

The list of "Famous People with ADHD" is long—and growing. All of the following people have publicly identified themselves as having ADHD. There are captains of industry such as Richard Branson (founder of Virgin Group). There are inventors and scientists such as Dean Kamen. There are entertainers such as Howie Mandel, Ryan Gosling, Emma Watson, Jim Carrey, Greta Gerwig, and David Blaine.

And there are many athletes, such as Simone Biles and Michael Phelps. Additionally, there is (unverifiable) speculation about historical figures who might have had ADHD, ranging from Leonardo da Vinci to Agatha Christie to Benjamin Franklin to Thomas Edison.

What *is* verifiable is that people with ADHD tend to see things in ways that people without ADHD sometimes miss. David Neeleman, the founder of JetBlue Airlines, said in a 2005 issue of ADDitude magazine, "If someone told me that you could be normal or you could continue to have ADHD, I would take ADHD . . . I knew I had strengths that other people didn't have, and my parents reminded me of them when my teachers didn't see them . . . I can distill complicated facts and come up with simple solutions. I can look out on an industry with all kinds of problems and say, 'How can I do this better?' " Similarly, Paul Orfalea, founder of Kinko's (now known as FedEx Office and Print Services), said, "Because I have a tendency to wander, I never spent much time in my office . . . If I had stayed in my office all the time, I would not have discovered all those wonderful ideas to help expand the business . . . My biggest advantage is that I don't get bogged down in the details because of my ADHD." These ADHDers took great ideas, combined them with high energy and a lack of patience for the unimportant parts, and formed new companies with innovative business plans—never allowing themselves to become inhibited by worrying too much about all the things that could go wrong.

There is a concept called **hyperfocus** that many ADHDers cherish. What is hyperfocus? Some ADHDers note that even though they have trouble focusing on many types of tasks, especially mundane boring tasks that everyone has to do to survive and stay healthy, they can at times get so focused on something that they tune out everything else. They become so absorbed that their world shrinks down to only the one task they are interested in, even to the point where it can become counterproductive and dangerous, lead to problems getting along with others, or interfere with doing other things they need to do. It is important to note that hyperfocus is not currently recognized as a sign or symptom of ADHD, although it might conceivably be in the future. There are those who believe it is specific to ADHD; others believe it is experienced by many people, not just ADHDers.

If there are these great upsides, then why would you treat ADHD? The idea of treatment is to keep the great parts while gaining more control over the difficult parts. As doctors we do not want to "zombify" our patients or make them just be "regular." We want to help them execute plans so that their excellent ideas come to fruition. We want to help them listen to other people so they can learn enough to take that information and do something fabulous with it. We want to give them control over their problematic impulses so that their energy can be directed into accomplishing what they truly want, rather than what happens to catch their eye in the moment.

So now that we've covered some basics about ADHD, how do you know if you have it? To find out, read on about diagnosis in Chapter 2!

CHAPTER 2

Diagnosis

Where and How to Get Help

In this chapter, you will learn:

- The right type of professional to diagnose your ADHD
- What your initial doctor's visit for ADHD will be like
- A brief history of ADHD diagnosis and current diagnostic criteria
- Surveys and tests that can help diagnose ADHD
- Whether you should get neuropsychological testing, a genetic test, or a brain scan for ADHD

Who Is the Right Professional to Diagnose My ADHD?

If you have a fever, a doctor might take a blood sample to check on the severity and source of infection. If you have a sharp pain in your arm after a bad fall, your doctor might order an X-ray or MRI to see if a bone is broken. But if you are frequently impulsive or distracted, there is no blood test or brain scan that can show whether you have ADHD. So how do doctors determine whether you have it?

Before we can even begin to answer that question, we first have to answer another: What kind of doctor is best qualified to diagnose ADHD? With many medical problems, the answer to this question is clearer. For example, if you have something wrong with your kidney, you go to a kidney specialist or **urologist**; if there is a problem with your heart, you go to a **cardiologist**. So what kind of doctor is an ADHD specialist?

Should You See a Psychologist (PhD) or a Physician (MD)?

In general, ADHD has to be diagnosed by a professional with a doctoral-level degree. There are two relevant professionals with very different degrees: **psychologists** and physicians. In general, psychologists focus more on **talk therapy** and behavioral interventions, whereas physicians focus more on prescribing medications (though some **psychiatrists** may also do talk therapy or other types of non-medication interventions). If you are open to taking medication to manage your ADHD, you almost certainly want to see a physician (or **nurse practitioner**—further information about this type of medical professional below). If, on the other hand, you really want to avoid taking medications and are strongly interested in non-medication strategies (such as **coaching** or talk therapy), a psychologist is almost certainly the better professional for you. In the end, many people wind up seeing both kinds of professionals to get all the help they need.

Doctoral-level psychologists have either a PhD (a degree that requires both clinical and research training) or a PsyD (a degree focused on clinical training only). Either type of psychologist can make an ADHD diagnosis and treat the condition. The chief criterion you should use to find the best psychologist to help you is how much ADHD they actually treat. Psychology encompasses the study and treatment of all human behavior, an extremely broad field. There are all sorts of subspecialists in psychology, so if you are looking for the most accurate diagnosis and best treatment for ADHD, then look for a psychologist for whom ADHD diagnosis and treatment is a big part of what they do. Does the psychologist say or advertise on their website that they work with a lot of clients who have ADHD? Do they appear to be very knowledgeable about and comfortable around this diagnosis? Or do they specialize in other areas of mental health? Look for one who focuses on ADHD as a main part of their practice and interest.

Most physicians have an MD (medical doctor) degree, though some may have a DO (doctor of osteopathy) degree; either an MD or a DO can specialize in some aspect of general practice (such as **internal medicine** or **family medicine**) or in a specialty (such as psychiatry or **neurology**). Most physicians would agree that ADHD is the domain of neurologists and psychiatrists. Even so, you may want to start the process of receiving medical assistance for your ADHD through your general practitioner, especially if you already have a good relationship with that doctor. Depending on their comfort with initiating ADHD diagnosis and treatment, your primary care doctor, who could be an **internist** or a **pediatrician**, should be able to refer you to an appropriate psychiatrist or neurologist to further your care.

A final word about professionals who can diagnose ADHD and prescribe medications: Many patients receive medical care from a **nurse practitioner** (NP) instead of from an MD or a DO. NPs are nurses who have received extra training so that they can diagnose and treat patients without a doctor's direct participation. Regulations around how NPs practice vary from state to state; in some states, NPs must work closely with a physician who supervises their practice, while in others, NPs can practice more independently. The type of NP most closely analogous to a psychiatrist is a **PMHNP** (psychiatric and mental health nurse practitioner). In general, NPs start out their careers with a bit less formal education in the foundational sciences underlying medicine than MDs or DOs. They also may have seen less of the inside of hospitals and of managing life-threatening illnesses during their early training—but they often make up for that with a wealth of hands-on experience, especially after they have been in practice for some time. Given the brief history of ADHD (see "A Brief History of ADHD Diagnosis" below), we advise that if you are faced with a choice between receiving care from an experienced PMHNP who has a professional interest in ADHD versus an MD or a DO who rarely diagnoses or treats the condition, you should certainly go with the more experienced and interested PMHNP.

What Will Your Initial Doctor's Visit for ADHD Be Like?

Of course, different types of professionals have different ways of going about things, so the answer to the question of what to expect for your first doctor visit about ADHD varies depending on which of the above options you go with. Individual providers may have their own idiosyncrasies as well. That said, there are some basic guidelines and commonalities.

As of the writing of this book, the diagnosis of ADHD is made chiefly through the process of interviewing the patient (you or your child), asking questions about current symptoms and history of symptoms, and direct observation of behavior in the visit. The medical professional will do a **mental status exam** as part of their diagnostic evaluation, which includes their impressions of how attentive, distractible, impulsive, and fidgety the patient is in conversation. This part of the evaluation will be invisible to you and/or your child: It happens as a matter of course and depends a lot on the clinical experience and expertise of the professional doing your evaluation. The evaluation will also include many specific questions about how you or your child function in different areas of life—that is, not just at work or at school, and not just at home in your family or personal life, but both. If the evaluation is for your child, then often a form will be given to the child's teacher to fill out as well. Moreover, if you or your child are not functioning as expected in some area, the professional will want to explore some alternate explanations for why this might be happening. For example, if the child being evaluated is flunking school, or if the adult is underperforming at work, is that because of inattention? Could it be from a learning disability like dyslexia? Or could it be something else such as a family crisis or a lack of sleep?

Here are some examples of questions you or your child might be asked as part of a typical ADHD evaluation:

- Do you have to work harder or longer than other people to get the same amount of work done? If so, what is it about your work style that takes such a long time?
- Do you make a lot of silly mistakes? We are not talking about mistakes based on "I don't understand something." We are talking about lots of careless "oopsie" mistakes such as copying a math problem down wrong or sending emails to the wrong people.
- Are you disorganized? Do you lose things a lot? Do you "leave a trail" and create messes for other people to clean up?
- Do you have trouble starting tasks, especially tasks that may be a bit boring but that are necessary for you to do, either at home or at work/school?
- When you do start a task, do you finish it? Or do you often get distracted in the middle of things and find you have started multiple projects but rarely complete any?
- Is it hard to stay with a task that requires sustained mental effort (such as reading a book)? When was the last time you read any book cover to cover?
- Can you get done what you need to get done, when you need to do it? (ADHD expert Russell Barkley, PhD, has observed that ADHD is not a disorder of not knowing what to do, it's a disorder of not doing what you know at the right times and places. It's a disorder of not being able to accomplish and finish the right activities at the right time.)
- Do you have trouble listening to people? Is your mind frequently thinking about other things when people are talking to you? Do you have to actively force yourself to listen

to people and not get distracted? Or is listening completely impossible?
- In conversations, do you often interrupt other people with your own thoughts, which may be unrelated to what they were just talking about? Do you receive a lot of negative feedback about this?
- Do you often put things off? Do you usually find yourself doing things at the last minute?
- Is it hard for you to prioritize and organize?
- Are you very forgetful? Do you remember your chores and your appointments?
- Are you very impulsive? Do you do or say things without thinking about them? A history of impulsiveness may include talking too much or being intrusive in social relationships ("butting in" where you don't belong). It may include having a hard time sitting still.
- Are you restless? Do you get up a lot—for example, in the middle of watching a TV show?

If you are an adult seeking to clarify a diagnosis for yourself, then the professional should also ask about how you functioned as a child (to the extent you can remember). Some questions they may ask are:

- Did your teachers complain that you were inattentive? Were you always daydreaming in class?
- Did you always finish projects at the last minute, or not at all?
- Did you have trouble doing what the rest of the class was doing when it was required of you?
- Did your teacher have to move you to prevent you from distracting students around you because of your behavior or because you were always talking?
- Were you a "troublemaker" in other ways?

If you are a parent who is seeking to clarify a diagnosis for your child, you may need to take into consideration how much you do for your child versus how much they do for themselves. This can sometimes complicate the answers to these questions. Your child may finish their homework, but only because you watch them like a hawk, monitor their homework time, and make them complete it. Your child may not lose things, but only because you are always organizing and putting things away for them. Many parents who have children with ADHD don't know where to set a limit in this regard. How much is the "right amount" to do for them? Sometimes well-meaning parents develop a relationship with their child in which the child doesn't do very much for themself. As a parent, you may feel you have little choice but to do this; after all, you're busy too! You can't wait a week for your child to finally put their laundry away or do their homework. But this can lead to bigger problems down the road, because sooner or later, your child will need to be able to organize their own tasks and meet deadlines independently. This can even happen in adult relationships. We've seen a similar dynamic between partners in relationships where one has ADHD and the other doesn't. The "slack" of the partner who has ADHD gets taken up by the one who doesn't. That works for the relationship until the person picking up the slack gets tired of doing so—inevitably, there will be misunderstandings leading to smoldering resentments and sometimes outright conflict.

A Brief History of ADHD Diagnosis

Before describing the current diagnostic criteria for ADHD, it may be helpful to put it in historical context. As with all neuropsychiatric conditions, the criteria for diagnosing ADHD reflect the society we live in. How we view and classify behavior (that is, what is considered "normal" and "abnormal") varies across cultures and changes over time. This is not just true for ADHD; it is true for all emotional and behavioral conditions. For example, what in modern industrialized nations is now typically classified as a mental illness called **major depression** was once called melancholia in Europe and the United States. In the past, people who suffered from periodic bouts of melancholia weren't necessarily considered to be ill—they were often viewed as being in keener contact with the spiritual or "infinite" realms.

When it comes to inattention and hyperactivity, there are written accounts in Europe of children with differences in these traits going back at least to the 1800s. In popular books, there were characters ("Fidgety Phil" and "Johnny Look In the Air") that, through the lens of today, appear to have ADHD. However, these books were written to serve as morality tales, not medical texts. The characters in question were not intended to demonstrate children who might benefit from a diagnosis and medical treatment; rather, they were meant to serve as examples of what happens when children are raised with poor moral standards and a lack of suitable parental discipline. By the early 1900s, a few physicians had started to write about a condition resembling ADHD in more clinical terms (though it went by completely different names), but even in these medical texts, the view persisted that such conditions represented a defect in "moral control." Such descriptions were generally applied only to school-aged children.

After the influenza pandemic of 1918, there was a pandemic of encephalitis lethargica (also known as the "sleeping sickness"). This was a mental illness (that is, a disruption in behavior) that was recognized as a brain disorder caused by the physiological aftermath of the flu. The 1918 influenza and subsequent encephalitis pandemic represented a watershed in Western medicine—they spurred more widespread adoption of the concept that all human behavior must be rooted in the anatomy and physiology of the brain. In the decade after 1918, there were children who had had influenza who were noted to have subsequent difficulties with hyperactivity. This was often attributed to encephalitis lethargica—that is, to the long-term after-effects of sleeping sickness. This led quite naturally to the view that maybe hyperactivity in children who did not have a history of influenza had similar root causes in the brain. This hyperactivity syndrome became known as hyperkinetic impulse disorder.

In general, the disorder we now call ADHD wasn't noticed by psychiatrists and psychologists for a long time. Instead, it first came to the attention of professionals who worked primarily with school-aged children—that is, educators and some pediatric specialists. The first physicians to get involved were **child neurologists**, who characterized the condition as minimal brain dysfunction to distinguish it from more severe or obvious conditions related to brain function such as spasticity, convulsions, or abnormally low IQ (for example, **cerebral palsy, epilepsy,** or **developmental delay**). Only later did **child psychiatrists** get involved. It wasn't until the early 1980s that the *Diagnostic and Statistical Manual of Mental Disorders* (DSM) incorporated the disorder into **psychiatry**. They also changed its name to highlight its inattentive features, calling it attention-deficit disorder (ADD) with (or without) hyperactivity.

It took more than another decade for psychiatry to formally consider that the childhood condition known as ADD might continue beyond adolescence and carry significant repercussions for adult patients. The most recent edition of the DSM, the DSM-5 (published in 2013), is the first edition to fully embrace the existence of adult ADHD by providing criteria clearly targeted only toward adult patients. It has also relabeled the disorder ADHD (instead of ADD) and has added specifiers to designate whether the condition involves predominantly inattentive features, predominantly hyperactive/impulsive features, or both combined.

What You Can Learn from the History of ADHD

ADHD is like many other mental disorders in that it has historically been stigmatized. In its earliest conception, what we now call ADHD was widely viewed as a moral disorder—"bad kids with bad parents"—and it is still viewed that way by many people. Both among the lay public and within professional circles, this legacy impacts diagnosis and treatment despite abundant scientific and clinical evidence that such a view is irrational and unfair.

Partly because of its history, there remains some confusion over which professionals "own" ADHD—that is, which specialists are "in charge" of diagnosing it. Even today, while most physicians would agree that ADHD is the province of neurologists and psychiatrists, many general neurologists and psychiatrists receive little formal training in its diagnosis and management and don't routinely screen for it or treat it, especially with regard to adult patients. Part of our motivation for writing this book is to help correct this situation.

ADHD, and particularly adult ADHD, is among the newest psychiatric diagnoses. Yet statistical information from the most reliable sources, including the Harvard Medical School and U.S. government agencies such as the **National Institutes of Health** (NIH), indicates that attention problems join mood and anxiety challenges as one of the top three major psychiatric challenges afflicting the adult population. Adults are now the fastest-growing population diagnosed with and treated for ADHD.

Current Diagnostic Criteria for ADHD

The professional doing the diagnosing, whether a neurologist, psychiatrist, other type of MD, NP, psychologist, or therapist, is generally considering whether their patient meets the "DSM criteria" for ADHD. The DSM-5 criteria for ADHD include the following potential symptoms (wording adapted from the DSM):

Inattention-Related Symptoms

- Makes careless mistakes in schoolwork, at work, or with other activities and often misses details.
- Has difficulty maintaining attention on tasks or play activities.

- Mind is frequently elsewhere when other people are talking.
- Tends to have difficulty finishing tasks related to schoolwork, chores, or workplace duties due to losing focus or becoming sidetracked.
- Is disorganized and messy.
- Procrastinates with non-preferred tasks.
- Loses or misplaces belongings frequently (for example, school materials, pencils, books, tools, wallets, keys, paperwork, eyeglasses, cellphone).
- Is easily distracted.
- Forgets tasks, responsibilities, and appointments.

Symptoms Related to Hyperactivity and Impulsivity

- Is fidgety and squirmy, frequently moving their hands or feet.
- Gets up from their chair in situations where being seated is the norm.
- Engages in inappropriate and/or unsafe running or climbing (adolescents or adults may be limited to feeling restless).
- Is louder and more raucous than those around them.
- Frequently "on the go," acting as if "driven by a motor."
- Talks more than expected in many situations.
- Impulsively "blurts out" comments or answers to questions.
- Has a hard time waiting in line.
- Tends to butt into conversations or games when they are not part of the group.

There are several major points to make about DSM criteria. First of all, as explained above, the criteria are created by a committee of experts, based on their professional experience and review of available scientific evidence, combined with considerable debate and inevitable compromises. As such, the criteria should never be viewed as absolute, especially as they change at least slightly (and sometimes more than slightly) with each new edition of the DSM. So the "official" symptom list and even the terminology for ADHD in the DSM-6 will likely have evolved from those described above on the basis of new clinical findings and research, just as the present criteria evolved from those in the previous edition (which barely mentioned the possibility of ADHD in adults), and just as those evolved from the edition before that (in which adult ADHD wasn't even alluded to). For example, based on current research and debate in the field, ADHD as defined in a future DSM might include a new symptom area, **affective dysregulation**, which refers to poor control of some emotional responses (such as crying very easily). This is a symptom that a lot of people with ADHD display, but it is not among the DSM-5 criteria.

> *Lola was always known as "the Tasmanian Devil" growing up. Her mother used to joke that she always knew where Lola had been in the house by the trail she left behind. In younger grades, Lola was frequently having to get up to "use the bathroom" or sharpen pencils. She always wanted to be first in line. She always seemed to have her hands on other people's stuff, and her dad sighed and said, "It makes me tired to even look at her" as she was "always moving," even while watching movies. She was very talkative, which was initially seen as cute, as she had a lot of interesting things to say. In early grade school, Lola was very popular, as she was a natural leader. However, in her teens she ran into increasing social issues. She blurted out comments about friends that they often did not appreciate. She became known as the person who always got told off by the teacher for talking or interrupting; other kids tired of her frequent disruptions to the class. She continued to lose her belongings, despite the items becoming more important and costly as she grew up, such as her phone or keys. She got kicked off the soccer team for repeatedly forgetting her cleats. She got kicked off the lacrosse team for forgetting to show up to practice.*

> *Lola became more and more withdrawn and easily upset. She spent a lot of time on her phone scrolling through YouTube. She felt the world was against her. She felt her teachers were not fair. She wanted to drive, but her parents were concerned about that as she had a hard time controlling her temper and was easily distracted. In fact, she became so irritable that anything would set her off. She would fly into a rage or start crying uncontrollably over a seemingly trivial comment or event.*

A cornerstone of current diagnosis is that the symptoms of ADHD affect people in more than one area of their life. A child does not have ADHD just because they have difficulty in one history class or with one teacher. Similarly, an adult with ADHD has symptoms in more than one area of their lives—they don't have it just because they hate their job or are bored with it; maybe they just need to get a different job! In the example about Lola above, her issues stretched over multiple years and arose in multiple situations.

On the other hand, a child who is very competitive and motivated to do well in school (whether they are self-motivated or motivated by pressure from parents) could compensate for ADHD symptoms, especially if they are bright enough. They may get the desired A's, but only because they work far harder than they should reasonably need to (for example, putting in double the number of homework hours and barely getting any sleep because they work more slowly due to distractibility). Similarly, many adults are much more functional in a highly structured work environment compared to when at home. We've had patients with ADHD who have careers as personal assistants: It's their job is to organize tasks for someone else. They can do this if they are paid for it and have learned to double-check their work and catch mistakes at the office. However, at home, where chores can be more easily put off without consequences, they fall way behind and things are a complete mess.

Another principle of diagnosis is that the symptoms of ADHD must have "no other reason." Again, rephrased from the DSM:

> Other neuropsychiatric disorders do not better explain the symptoms. (For example, anxiety could explain restlessness, depression could explain poor motivation, and **schizophrenia** could explain poor attention.)

As we will describe in greater detail in Chapter 5, there are many other conditions, both psychiatric and medical, that can mimic ADHD. To take one medical example, if a person has severe **obstructive sleep apnea**, a condition where sleep is not restful or restorative, they may have attentional difficulties that look just like ADHD, but these symptoms are secondary to their brain not functioning well because it never gets a good night's rest—and that's *not* ADHD. Another common cause of inattention is **major depression**. In fact, poor motivation, being unable to get work done, and poor concentration are among the primary symptoms of depression. So how can you tell the difference? Well, among other differences, depression and other **mood disorders** tend to be cyclical, whereas ADHD is constant. If your inattentive symptoms come and go and tend to occur in the context of high stress and low mood, the cause is more likely to be a mood disorder and not ADHD (although it could be a combination of both; one could be making the other worse). Additionally, if you have symptoms of ADHD but also drink alcohol or smoke cannabis daily, it's going to be very difficult to tease apart how much of your attentional difficulties are due to ADHD versus chronic use of substances that independently impair concentration, productivity, energy levels, task management, and motivation.

The DSM also stipulates that symptoms must be severe enough to impact daily life in a very meaningful way:

> There is clear evidence that the symptoms interfere with, or reduce the quality of, social, school, or work functioning.

This is an extremely important point, not just about ADHD, but about every psychiatric condition. Many people read, see a video, or hear about diagnostic criteria for a psychiatric disorder on the internet or social media and think: "Oh, that's me! I must have that disorder!" This is good news in some ways—for one thing, it helps decrease stigma and increase social acceptance around these conditions. However, this type of self-diagnosis can be very deceptive. Part of the problem is that ADHD is a **quantitative,** as opposed to a **qualitative,** diagnosis. That is, people with ADHD aren't fundamentally different from anybody else in terms of their behavior; they are simply at the extreme end of the normal distribution of inattentiveness, impulsivity, and fidgetiness (Figure 2.1).

What this means is that, if you read the DSM-5 criteria for ADHD, you are likely to relate to the symptoms whether you have ADHD or not, because *everybody* is inattentive, impulsive, and/or hyperactive *sometimes*. That is, the diagnostic criteria for ADHD describe everybody to some degree—people with ADHD are simply more that way than is typical. Everybody occasionally misplaces their car keys. Everybody has challenges getting started on boring tasks. Everybody sometimes has trouble sticking to and finishing projects. Everybody

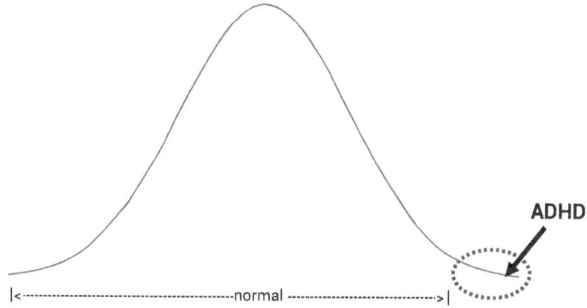

FIGURE 2.1 Graph of the distribution of inattentive, impulsive, or hyperactive symptoms in a population. Most people fall somewhere near the central bulge of the "normal distribution" or "bell curve." Those with ADHD lie at the extreme end of symptom severity.

has been bored to tears in a work meeting before. Everybody is occasionally diverted and distracted by their smartphone. Everybody has made the faux pas of interrupting someone with a non sequitur in conversation. Everybody fidgets sometimes, or occasionally gets up to walk around because they just can't sit still anymore. And, by the way, nearly everybody's significant other (if they've been together long enough) complains that they "never listen."

So the key question is not whether these symptoms ever happen to you (of course they do; you're human!) but whether they happen so much and so often that they cause significant problems in your personal or professional life. Have you lost jobs or been passed over for promotion because of your challenges with task management? Have people in your personal life cut you off because they are so sick of you interrupting them in conversation? Is the bank about to foreclose on your home because you keep forgetting to pay your mortgage, even though you have the money to do so? Is the government about to break down your door because you haven't filed your tax returns for the past 10 years—not because you've been trying to avoid paying taxes but because you can't get your act together to complete your tax forms? Are those forms sitting in one of the innumerable piles of paper littering your desk, among scattered sticky notes and uncompleted "to-do" lists?

Tests That Help Diagnose ADHD

There are no scientifically or clinically valid **blood tests**, **genetic tests**, or **brain scans** available for ADHD. Yet you may have heard of "ADHD testing." What does this mean?

The term "ADHD testing" is often used a bit loosely. One common type of ADHD "test" is actually not a test but a survey of questions for you to answer about your symptoms (or for someone else to fill out about you or your child). These survey "instruments" may be given on paper and answered with pen or pencil, or, increasingly, delivered and answered electronically. They are then scored numerically. There are many varieties of these survey instruments that go by different names and acronyms—for example, the ASRS, CAARS, NICHQ Vanderbilt, Connors, WURS, and ADHD-RS. It is beyond the scope of this book to go into detail about any of them in particular, but we will make a few general points.

Whether we are talking about adult or childhood ADHD, the survey instruments can be divided into two basic categories: self-rated and observer-rated. As these names suggest, self-rated surveys are lists of questions a patient answers about themselves, whereas observer-rated surveys are lists of questions somebody who knows a patient well answers about them. When children are being evaluated for ADHD, observer-rated surveys are the norm. Typically, these are filled out independently both by a parent and by the child's teachers. The reason why observer-rated surveys are the norm for children is simply that children are not thought to be capable of reliably answering a survey about themselves—although we have to point out we're not sure this has ever actually been clinically tested.

For adults who are being evaluated for ADHD, it is most common to have them do one of the self-rated survey instruments. That said, for adults as much as for children, it can be extremely useful to ask another person who knows them well to complete an observer-rated survey about their symptoms as well. This type of collateral information can be extremely helpful when considering the diagnosis, and it often leads to insightful discussions with the patient about their symptom challenges and how they view themself compared to how they are seen by the important people in their lives.

The first important point to make about all these surveys is that they are subjective and that none of them measure anything biological or behavioral about the person being evaluated for ADHD. The survey is scored based on what the person *says* about themselves (or, in the case of an observer-rated survey, what someone else says about them), and these answers are then compared to what a normal sample of people of the same gender and age similarly *say* about themselves (or others in the case of the observer-rated surveys). So these survey instruments don't measure attention, impulsivity, or hyperactivity directly. Instead, they measure what you *say* (or what someone who knows you well says) about your attention, impulsivity, and hyperactivity, compared to what a sample of other people *say* in response to the same sorts of questions.

These results can still be helpful insofar as they do quantitatively tell you where you stand compared to most other people in terms of what you believe about yourself and your possible ADHD symptoms, provided you answered all the questions as accurately as you could. But even if you do so, the test may still be skewed. A person concerned about ADHD is likely to selectively recall incidents that support the diagnosis. There is a well-defined psychological concept called **recall bias** that describes this phenomenon: Unintentionally, people tend to remember the times in their life where they were the most inattentive or hyperactive, and don't recall the times where they functioned well.

Some of the survey instruments include a "consistency index" that tries to show if the person filling out the questions is giving consistent answers, even if the questions are asked a little differently. The idea is to make sure that the patient has clear and steady concerns and that they truly know about living with ADHD, rather than just randomly faking answers about things that they don't actually experience. But ironically, people who attempt to "fake" a diagnosis on such surveys actually tend to be very consistent in how they answer the questions. In other words, "fakers" tend to have very low "inconsistency indexes," and their tests are read as "valid." A high inconsistency index doesn't necessarily indicate the person who answered the survey was trying to fake the diagnosis; it could indicate that they didn't understand all of the questions or that they felt put off by the wording of some of the questions.

Are there other, more objective, tests for ADHD? In short, the answer is *yes*.

Recently, a brain wave test called the Neuropsychiatric EEG-Based Assessment Aid (NEBA) system was approved by the U.S. Food and Drug Administration (FDA) for helping diagnose ADHD in children and adolescents (it is not FDA approved for adults). It looks at a person's electrical brain waves to see if there is a pattern that might support a diagnosis of ADHD. Importantly, it has not been approved as a stand-alone test for ADHD. Instead, it is supposed to be used along with a doctor's clinical impressions from the office visit to help make the diagnosis more secure by providing a relevant **biomarker** for the disorder. The NEBA system, however, is not widely used currently.

Another type of objective test for ADHD is a computerized test that assesses attention, distractibility, and sometimes fidgetiness or hyperactivity. It is generically called a **continuous performance task**, though there are several varieties, including the T.O.V.A., CPT-3, and QB Test. These tests are all conceptually very similar in that they ask the test-taker to click a button or hit a spacebar on their keyboard every time they either hear a certain repeated tone, see a repeated shape, or see a letter on their screen, but not to hit the button or spacebar at other times or in other conditions. The duration of the tests is typically between 10 and 20 minutes. The test is designed to be long and quite boring, and that is the whole point: The test-taker is being asked to pay attention for over 10 minutes while repeating a very boring task. This is difficult for anybody, let alone somebody with ADHD. The computer collects data about how often the test-taker pushes the button correctly versus incorrectly, how often they responded as quickly as they were supposed to, how consistent they were with this response time, and (sometimes) how fidgety they were throughout the test-taking session. Again, this information gets compared to similar data from a sample of people of the same gender and age as the test-taker who took an identical test.

An advantage of these types of computerized tests is that they are more objective than the survey instruments described before. The computerized tests do measure actual behavior; that is, how well you are able to pay attention for about 10 to 20 minutes while doing a repetitive computerized task. But that still doesn't make them perfect. For one thing, it is possible to "cheat" on these tests by purposely doing poorly (although that is sometimes obvious based on the pattern of responses). More importantly, these tests are highly artificial in what they are asking a person to do. Focusing for 10 to 20 minutes on something that is happening on a computer screen is not the same as focusing during a lecture or business meeting, doing your taxes, or resisting your impulse to interrupt someone in conversation. So the tests are certainly measuring something behavioral, but that may or may not be a good measure of the most relevant symptoms of ADHD in individual cases. Moreover, the very fact that these tests are computerized may backfire in certain cases. Although the makers of the tests claim this is not the case, we have had patients who have obvious signs and symptoms of ADHD based on all other aspects of their evaluation but who love to play videogames competitively and who did very well on the continuous performance task they were asked to do. When we asked them about the test, they said, "I loved it! It was like a videogame. I worked really hard to beat it." As noted above, the design of the test is that it is *supposed* to be challenging by being *boring*—so what does it mean when someone with attentional difficulties everywhere else in their life "aces" such a test because they are preconditioned to love playing simple screen games?

Do I (or Does My Child) Need Neuropsychological Testing for ADHD?

The type of computerized test described above, a continuous performance task, is an office-based test that can be done for ADHD but that is also often included as part of a much broader battery of behavioral tests referred to as **neuropsychological testing**. These tests are conducted by qualified clinical psychologists and take several hours to complete. They are also often quite expensive. Beyond the continuous performance task test itself, which is specifically designed to help diagnose ADHD, is it necessary to get a full neuropsychological test battery?

The answer is that it depends on what problem you are trying to solve and, often, on how old you are. Usually, neuropsychological testing is most relevant for school-aged children. If your child is struggling academically, it can often be unclear exactly what the source of the problem is, but it is crucial to figure it out. For example, if your child isn't reading well, could it be because of ADHD? After all, if you can't concentrate on what you are reading, you will not be able to absorb its meaning. However, the cause could also be **dyslexia**. Dyslexia is a problem of decoding—that is, quickly and automatically processing what letters are and how they are linked to particular sounds. Dyslexia is just one example of a learning disability—a condition that makes it more difficult for someone to achieve a specific skill by the age that most people are able to learn it. Dyslexia is also an example of a language-based learning disability. There are other types of well-defined learning disabilities—for example, those that affect a person's ability to learn math, or to learn visuospatial skills. For a child who is struggling in school, it is critical to determine what the most limiting issue is for the child, because knowing this will dictate the best course of action to help them cope with the problem. Of course, many children have multiple learning disabilities—for example, dyslexia is often **comorbid** (that is, it occurs together) in kids with ADHD. Treating some learning disabilities involves providing coaching on specific skills, such as helping a child with dyslexia learn to identify letters properly, or focusing on reading comprehension or math drills with a child who has specific problems in those areas. In contrast, treating the attentional part of learning (ADHD) requires focusing on other specific coping strategies (for instance, turning off distractions, or simply helping them view reading as important). It may also mean the child needs to take a medication to improve their attention and to decrease distractibility while in class.

Testing for learning disabilities is often done in schools. Schools usually have master's-level professionals who do this. These professionals can do limited testing for learning disabilities to see whether or not the child in question is eligible for special help through the school district. They are often located onsite so that the child can be observed in the classroom and so "on-the-ground" observations can be made. Such testing is often initiated by parents meeting with teachers and the principal or other school administrators to request an **IEP** evaluation. IEP stands for **individual education plan**. If your child needs an IEP, it means they need support that involves specialized instruction. The school is required to run appropriate tests to see if your child qualifies for an IEP.

Under a federal law originally called the Rehabilitation Act of 1973, but since reauthorized under the Individuals with Disabilities Education Act (IDEA), all school districts are required to provide free and appropriate public education (FAPE) to each qualified student with a disability who is in the school district's jurisdiction. Whether your child goes to a public or private school, if you live in a school district, you are eligible to receive some services from that district if your child needs extra help to get an "appropriate" education. Section 504 of the Rehabilitation Act refers to programs and activities that receive federal financial assistance from the U.S. Department of Education; as such, a "504 plan" commonly refers to accommodations kids receive from their school district that do not require special kinds of teaching. Examples might include an accommodation to turn in homework late or to take extra time on tests.

> *Cindy is an 8-year-old girl whose teachers have contacted her parents because she is falling behind in class. During class, she often seems to be distracted; her teacher notes that this seems to be most obvious when they are working on reading skills but may happen at other times too. Cindy is lagging behind the*

> other children in reading, both in terms of fluency with reading aloud and in terms of her ability to comprehend what she reads. Her teacher is concerned that Cindy is becoming self-conscious about this as well, leading to an avoidance of reading. Cindy's handwriting is also below what is expected for her age. Math is relatively better, but she tends to make silly mistakes and race through her work.
>
> After a meeting at the school with the teacher, Cindy's parents, and the principal of the school, it was agreed that IEP testing be done. An educational psychologist tested Cindy's academic abilities. Everybody met to discuss the results. Cindy was far enough behind to qualify for specialized help at the school. The IEP clarified what that help was to be: Cindy would get individual help for reading and writing. The IEP did not say whether or not she had dyslexia but did give a plan to help her with reading and writing skills, and defined expectations and goals about how fast she was expected to progress.

In the psychology community, there are specialized psychologists called **educational psychologists** who do **educational psychological testing** to test how people (usually children) learn. An educational psychologist may conduct tests on memory, reading, math, and other areas of academic achievement. They will test IQ. They will also administer survey instruments to parents and teachers, including the ones mentioned above for ADHD, and process the results. Neuropsychologists have even more training than educational psychologists and may do additional (and different) tests to assess which areas of a person's brain may be impaired. In contrast to the tests focused only on ADHD, which can be completed in as little as a few minutes to as long as 1 to 2 hours, school-based testing, educational psychologists' testing, or neuropsychological testing can take many hours. As described above, the school district is obliged by law to provide some of this testing for free if there is a reasonable suspicion a child needs extra help. Testing done outside of the school district is often more comprehensive. Sometimes it is covered (or, more likely, partly covered) by health insurance plans, but most often you will need to pay for it out of pocket, and it can run up to several thousands of dollars.

None of this additional testing is needed for a diagnosis of ADHD to be made. But if there is a suspicion that other learning disabilities such as dyslexia may be present in a school-aged child, getting this type of full test battery done is critical, because each specific learning disability must be addressed for the child to succeed in school—especially as struggles in school can cascade into other lifelong consequences.

Should I (or My Child) Get a Genetic Test or Brain Scan for ADHD?

In Chapter 3, we will discuss what is known about the biology of ADHD. For now, suffice it to say that while scientific progress is always being made, current science related to ADHD is extremely incomplete. A question that our patients often ask us is whether a blood test, genetic test, or brain scan can help make the diagnosis. The short answer is *no*.

Genetic Testing

We discuss this more in Chapter 3. Here, we will simply say that while progress is always being made and we have hopes for the future, for now routine genetic testing cannot reveal whether someone has ADHD. There is also genetic testing being marketed to optimize medication treatment. We will discuss this further in Chapter 6 where we discuss ADHD medications, but once again, for now we will note that this type of testing is not recommended by any official professional organizations (for example, the American Psychiatric Association or American Medical Association) nor by the FDA for this purpose.

Brain Scans

There are companies marketing brain scans such as "Brain SPECT" to diagnose ADHD and other neuropsychiatric disorders. If you think you have ADHD (or another psychiatric condition) and are considering paying for such services, we urge caution—and recommend saving your money. As physicians, we always favor gathering objective information about your medical condition. As scientists, we have great hopes for progress that may one day make brain imaging useful for ADHD diagnosis and treatment. Unfortunately, at this time there is no valid scientific or clinical basis for claims that individuals with ADHD can be better diagnosed, or their treatment optimized, through the use of any kind of brain scan. If you wish to understand more about the underlying biology regarding this, please read Chapter 3.

We certainly agree it would be great if your doctor could scan your brain or your DNA, tell you what your psychiatric diagnosis is, and determine the best medication for you to take. That day may come, but for now, it remains science fiction. There is no test or scan available today that can reveal in sufficient resolution these facts about you or your loved one with ADHD. In the future, eye tracking tests or other developing technologies may be helpful.

In summary, diagnosis for ADHD can be difficult because it is heavily subjective. The diagnosis of ADHD is *not* based on a unique set of behaviors or symptoms that people without ADHD never experience. Rather, it is based on a person's behavior being at the extreme end of normal for inattention, impulsivity, and hyperactivity—so much so that it causes very significant problems in their life. While there are clinically validated symptom surveys and some behavioral tests that can help support a diagnosis, there is currently no way to diagnose ADHD based purely on a test result. There is also not just one type of professional who can make the diagnosis, and different professionals may take different stances in any given patient case. As progress is continually being made, we hope that in the future there will be clear biological tests to help better define and diagnose ADHD.

CHAPTER 3

What Causes ADHD?

Biology

In this chapter, you will learn:

- Whether brain structures and brain growth are different in ADHD
- What scientists understand about different brain function in ADHD
- Brain chemicals involved in ADHD
- The role of genes and heredity in ADHD
- Why genetic tests and brain scans don't work to diagnose ADHD

A Permission Slip for Our Readers

This chapter summarizes current biological science relevant to ADHD. It is a bit technical for some readers, so it's perfectly fine to skip it if you wish. The science of ADHD gets complicated very quickly, so don't worry if you can't follow all of it, especially on just one reading. Although we have faith that it will eventually pay off and one day prove useful, at this time the state of the art in the neuroscience of ADHD is incomplete and not very useful for practical treatment and management decision-making. There is still far too much that scientists and doctors don't understand about how the brain works and about human genetics to make this type of information useful for diagnosis or treatment.

Are Any Brain Structures Abnormal or Different in ADHD?

Thoughts, emotions, and behaviors are largely the product of a single organ in your body: the brain. This may seem obvious to most people now, but it wasn't always accepted wisdom. Aristotle, for example, believed that the heart was the seat of consciousness and that the brain was primarily an organ for dispersing heat, like a radiator. Traditionally, and even today, many cultures around the world localize some emotions and impulses to the heart, gut, or other bodily parts and organs. Western science has accepted that the brain is the organ where thoughts and emotions are generated, but it still can't fully explain how this happens. The connection between the brain's structure and its function is significantly more complicated than the connection between structure and function for any other organ in the body. That said, we'll cover some basic information relevant to ADHD in this chapter.

The first point to make is that, in a significant sense, the human brain isn't just a single organ with a single function. It is composed of different regions specialized to help generate different aspects of our mental life. These brain regions communicate with each other. The connections between brain regions are often referred to as **brain circuits** or **brain networks** to compare them to computer circuits or electronic networks—but the circuits in your brain are organized very differently and use a different logic than the ones in a computer or any other electronic gadget humans have created. Scientists don't yet fully understand how the brain is organized, let alone how this organization is impacted by a mental condition like ADHD. Scientists can take pictures of the brain using brain imaging (for example, CT [**computed tomography**] and MRI [**magnetic resonance imaging**] scans) to examine how much individual variation there is in the size and structure of different brain regions in people with ADHD. They may see differences in shapes of the regions but will still not understand how the regions all work together.

Some brain areas in people with ADHD seem to be smaller than in those without ADHD. Those differences are likely involved in the cause of ADHD; however, it's also possible that the reverse is true: that having ADHD causes these brain areas to become smaller. It's important to note that even though these brain areas are statistically a tiny bit different in people with ADHD when you look at many of them together, there is a huge amount of variation and overlap with the "normal" population. This has critical implications for whether you can use this type of information for diagnostic purposes. (Spoiler alert: You can't! See further information in "Diagnostic Implications of Brain Anatomy and Brain Growth Studies" below.) Some brain areas identified as being slightly smaller in these types of brain imaging studies include:

- The **corpus callosum**—a bundle of **fibers** connecting the left and right hemispheres of the brain that facilitates long-distance and bilateral communication between many brain regions
- Several components of the **limbic system**, including the:
  - *Nucleus accumbens*, which is involved in motivation and rewards
  - *Amygdala,* which is involved in negative reinforcement and associated emotional reactions such as fear and revulsion; also a component of the **salience network** (see "What About Differences in Brain Function?" below)
  - *Hippocampus*, which is involved in learning and memory; often considered a component of the **default**

mode network (see "What About Differences in Brain Function?" below)
- Several components of the **basal ganglia**, including the:
  - *Caudate*, which helps in the planning of voluntary movement, and also in processing many other types of information
  - *Putamen*, which helps in preparation and execution of movement, including speech, as well as in some aspects of learning and rewards
- The **temporal cortex**, the outer layer of the bottom-most lobe of the cerebral cortex (extending sideways roughly underneath the ears)—involved (among other things) in processing auditory and some visual information, as well as **affect** and emotions and in some types of external reward. Different areas of the temporal lobe are components of both the **default mode network** and the **task-positive network** (also known as the **central executive network** or **attention network**—it will be discussed further in "What About Differences in Brain Function?" below).

This is not a definitive list of all the brain regions implicated in ADHD. Such a list cannot be provided, because brain imaging of ADHD is an area of active scientific research. In fact, there is extensive disagreement among scientists and across research studies about which brain areas are structurally different in ADHD.

There are, nevertheless, a few important points to keep in mind: (1) There are many regions in the brain, and they are widely distributed, and (2) each region includes structures, such as the corpus callosum, considered to be primarily involved in communication between different areas on both sides of the brain. If we consider both of these facts together, it becomes clear that ADHD is *not* a disorder of a single brain area, but that it results from the interplay between many different brain regions.

Differences in Brain Growth in ADHD

Another way to consider brain structure and how it relates to ADHD is by examining how the brain changes over a lifetime. As we will discuss further in Chapter 10, the brains of children are different from the brains of adults. Naturally, your brain grows and develops along with the rest of you. Is this growth somehow different in children with ADHD? This is a great question, but one that is difficult to answer by doing research because of the number of brain scans you'd have to repeat and compare over years and years in many children both with and without ADHD. Impressively, some scientists at the National Institutes of Health (NIH) have embarked on this ambitious type of research and have succeeded in gathering some evidence for the hypothesis that brain growth is a little different in kids with ADHD. Specifically, these researchers have found that, on average, brain areas responsible for executive functioning (the decision-making part of the brain) may develop a bit more slowly than brain areas responsible for generating emotions and impulses in children and adolescents with ADHD compared to those without the diagnosis.

Diagnostic Implications of Brain Anatomy and Brain Growth Studies

It is critically important to note that while scientific studies like those mentioned above have identified statistically significant differences in the sizes of certain brain regions in children, adolescents, and adults with ADHD, these differences are extremely tiny and heavily overlap with normal variation found in people who don't have ADHD. What this means is that this information, as interesting as it may be from a purely scientific point of view, cannot be used to distinguish someone with ADHD from someone without ADHD. In other words, if we did a brain scan on you and got a result showing that your amygdala is a little smaller than average, that *could* be consistent with ADHD, but it is *also* perfectly consistent with normal variation. There is no way to distinguish between these two alternatives. Simply put, there is no way, at present, to do a diagnostic brain scan on an individual to determine if they do or do not have ADHD.

What About Differences in Brain Function?

Now that we've discussed differences in brain structure, what about differences in brain activity? Scientific researchers can examine the activity of brain regions using specialized scans designed just for that, such as a **PET** (**positron emission tomography**) or **SPECT** (**single photon emission computed tomography**) scan. But does this type of imaging provide any insight into ADHD?

As with the anatomical brain research mentioned in the previous section, this is an area of active scientific research, and as yet, there is no consensus about the findings in ADHD. At best, this type of research has generated some interesting theories that are worth mentioning because they may give you an additional framework for understanding what is going on in the disorder. One of the most prominent theories about brain activity in ADHD involves the ability to switch between different brain networks: specifically, the **default mode network** (DMN) versus the **task-positive network** (TPN). In simple terms, the DMN is a set of interconnected brain regions (commonly thought to include the **dorsomedial prefrontal cortex, posterior cingulate cortex/precuneus, angular gyrus**, and sometimes the hippocampus) that is normally active when you are not focused on anything in particular (for example, daydreaming, musing, thinking creatively, being "in the flow"). In contrast, the TPN (also known as the CEN or attention network, with minor technical differences) is a network of other interconnected brain areas that are more active when you are focused on accomplishing a task or thinking about something specific.

Activity in the DMN is normally "anticorrelated" with activity in the TPN (and other networks involved in generating attention), meaning that when the TPN turns on, the DMN should turn off, and vice versa. The **DMN interference model** of ADHD posits that in ADHD, these networks are improperly connected such that they are more often active at the same time. The result is what we observe in people with ADHD: They are more easily distracted, they daydream more, and it is more difficult for them to pay attention.

There is a slightly more elaborate model called the **triple network model** that incorporates yet a third brain network, the salience network (SN). This network includes some other brain regions, like the amygdala (see the bulleted list in "Are Any Brain Structures Abnormal or Different in ADHD?"). It activates when something important happens in your environment that should capture your attention (such as if there were a tiger lurking in the bushes—or, more likely today, if the strict and scary teacher at the front of your class is explaining an important math concept). The idea is that the SN should tell your brain when it's time to switch modes from the DMN to an attention network like the TPN, but in ADHD the SN doesn't work properly.

None of these models have been scientifically proven to be correct or critical in ADHD. The DMN interference model and the triple network model are best thought of as hypotheses that help illustrate how we can understand ADHD based on what scientists have worked out so far about how the brain works.

What Brain Chemicals Are Involved in ADHD?

Differences in brain function do not just arise from the different sizes, shapes, or activities of brain regions or from differences in the circuits and networks between them. Another important factor is the chemicals involved in communicating between individual brain cells (**neurons**) that make up all brain regions. These chemicals are called

neurotransmitters. Neurons, in general, are shaped like microscopic trees with a stem and branches that connect them to other neurons, sometimes over quite long distances, terminating in special communication zones called **synapses**. Neurotransmitters are released at these synapses to allow neurons to communicate with each other. The function of a neurotransmitter may be to tell the next neuron to "fire"—that is, to send an electrical signal down its branches. This electrical signal gets converted into new neurotransmitter signals at the next set of synapses, thereby transmitting signals to the next neuron(s) down the line, and so on.

For each neurotransmitter, there are many different **neurotransmitter receptors**. Neurotransmitter receptors are on the receiving end of the synapse and tell the next neuron in line what to do in response to the neurotransmitter (see Figure 3.1). While some neurotransmitter signals tell the next neuron in line to fire, others may tell the next neuron in line not to fire, some may just change the tendency to fire, and others may do far more complex things. The bottom line is that a neurotransmitter signal released by a neuron can cause different responses depending on the receptors present in the receiving neuron. But it gets even more complicated: The response of the receiving neuron also depends on other contextual factors, such as (1) whether the signal was received once or many times in rapid

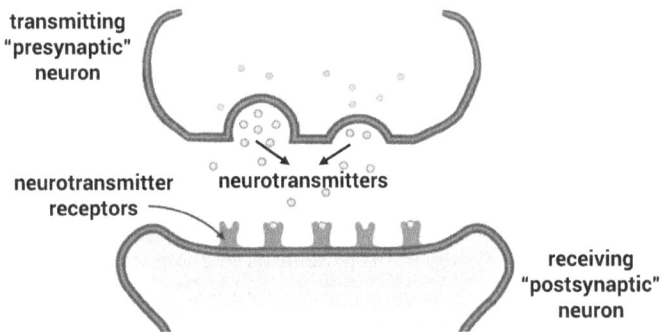

FIGURE 3.1 Simplified diagram of a synapse.

succession, (2) the amount of time since the receiving neuron last fired, and (3) what other types of signals were present around the same time at other synapses on the receiving neuron's other branches.

Why is all of this important? Some people have the impression that ADHD or any other mental disorder is as simple as "I have too little dopamine/serotonin" or that there is a "chemical imbalance" of some kind. Such explanations are tempting, chiefly because of the way they fit in with what little we understand about how medications for these conditions work. However, at best they are vast oversimplifications of a very complicated picture that scientists don't yet understand; at worst, they are simply incorrect.

So what does all this mean for ADHD? There are a handful of major neurotransmitters and several dozen minor ones; depending on whom you ask, the total number of neurotransmitters in the human brain ranges from 40 to over 100. Based chiefly on how medications for ADHD work, the two most important neurotransmitters in ADHD are thought to be **dopamine** and **norepinephrine**.

Chemically speaking, dopamine and norepinephrine are structurally very closely related **monoamines**. In fact, your body uses a single **enzyme** to synthesize norepinephrine directly from dopamine. To refer back to the previous section on brain anatomy, each of these neurotransmitters is made by a small number of neurons whose cell bodies are located in one of two small brain regions located near the connection of your brain to your spine (the brainstem). But even though these neurons are the sole source of these two neurotransmitters, they have long projections that reach out into many other brain areas (Figure 3.2). The result is that even though dopamine and norepinephrine are made by neurons whose cell bodies are located in small clumps near your brainstem, these chemicals are released widely to affect the activity of neurons in many other brain areas, circuits, and networks.

What do these two neurotransmitters do? **Dopamine** is involved in regulating cognition, sensory perception, attention, and motivation (reward). Looking at the diagram shown in Figure 3.2 and comparing

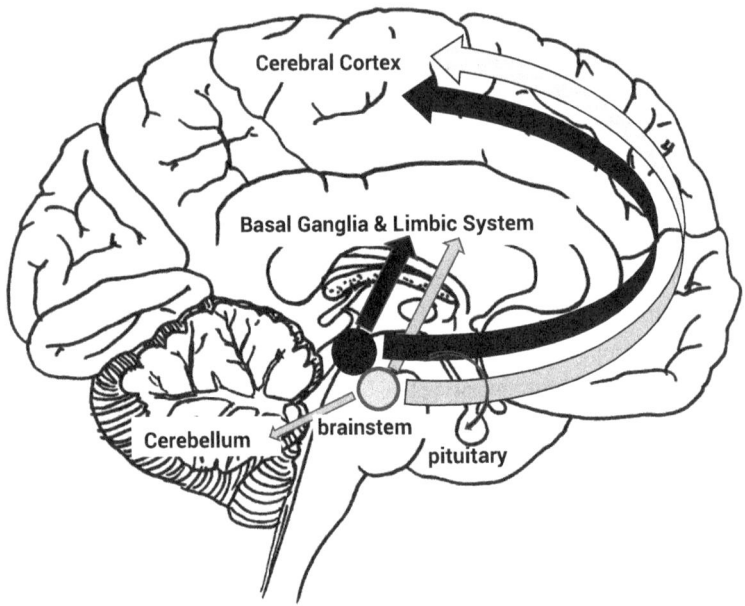

FIGURE 3.2 Dopamine (dark) and norepinephrine (light) projections in the human brain.

it to the earlier list of brain areas implicated in ADHD, you can see that dopamine produced in the brainstem is released in both the basal ganglia and the limbic system deep in the center of your brain. This makes some sense, as these same brain areas have some minor anatomical differences in people with ADHD based on brain imaging studies. Dopamine is also released in more superficial areas such as the cerebral cortex, especially near the front of your brain. These areas are implicated in the TPN, or attention networks, discussed in the previous sections about brain activity differences in ADHD.

Norepinephrine is chemically closely related to both dopamine and epinephrine, which you may know better by its other name: **adrenaline**. Just as adrenaline revs up your body whenever it needs to move, norepinephrine (also known as **noradrenaline**) revs up your brain whenever it needs to pay attention. In simple terms, norepinephrine is the neurotransmitter that tells many different parts of your brain, "Hey, wake up! Be on the alert! Something important is coming!" Accordingly, levels of norepinephrine are generally highest in the morning and lowest at night, but can also be released in response to stress or when you are actively doing something. As you can see in Figure 3.2, norepinephrine is released in many brain areas involved in the attention network or TPN (see previous section on brain activity models), such as the cerebral cortex. It is also released in the cerebellum, which is primarily involved in coordinating movement.

This discussion helps us understand why having low dopamine or norepinephrine signaling in your brain could contribute to ADHD, but it's also important to note that both of these neurotransmitters do many other things and are implicated in other neuropsychiatric disorders and behaviors beyond those we've described. For example, dopamine is a major neurotransmitter in the reward circuitry of the brain and is therefore a critical player in all forms of addiction. Low levels of dopamine are linked to conditions such as depression and dementia, whereas high levels are linked to **psychosis**, such as in schizophrenia. Dopamine is also critical in the brain circuitry controlling movement; because of this, damage to the dopamine-producing cells in the brainstem is at the center of Parkinson disease (which is characterized in part by muscle rigidity and loss of voluntary movement). Further, having too much dopamine relative to another neurotransmitter is central to Huntington chorea (which is characterized by a lot of extra movement that is difficult to control). As if that were not enough, dopamine (via regulation of the hormone prolactin released from the pituitary) is also the neurotransmitter that regulates milk production in nursing mothers. As for norepinephrine, besides its role in ADHD, low levels are linked to depression, while both high and low levels are linked to anxiety and **panic** disorders.

Hope for the Future: Combining Brain Anatomy with Brain Chemistry

There is a technology called a **DAT** (*do*p*a*mine *t*ransporter) **scan** that uses **radiolabeled tracers** to detect brain areas that are actively using dopamine. Scientists are doing research using DAT to monitor the activity of dopamine transporters in different brain regions in people with and without ADHD, both at baseline and while taking medication. While not yet ready for widespread clinical use, this approach could lead to some interesting advancements in the future.

The Role of Heredity (Genes) in ADHD

One reason we know that ADHD has a biological basis is because it tends to run in families. In general, if you have a first-degree relative (that is, a parent, child, or full sibling) who has ADHD, your own likelihood of also having ADHD is several times higher than in the general population. In some studies, the increased likelihood of having ADHD is as much as eight times higher in first-degree relatives of those already diagnosed with ADHD. The overall **heritability** of ADHD, which refers to the likelihood of having a disorder that comes from genetics, is around 74%, similar to other major heritable mental health conditions such as schizophrenia or bipolar disorder. This is important for several reasons. If you are an adult newly diagnosed with ADHD and you have children, you should consider the possibility that one or more of your children may have it as well. If, in retrospect, you feel your life might have gone better had you been diagnosed and treated earlier, you should consider having your kids evaluated, too. Similarly, if you are an adult whose child has recently been diagnosed with ADHD, you might want to consider whether you have similar problems and might benefit from treatment.

It is important to note that although ADHD tends to run in families, the subtypes or "presentations" of ADHD do not run true in the same way. That is, the predominance of hyperactive-impulsive or inattentive traits do not seem to be the same within a given family. To put this plainly: In most families where ADHD is present, one family member may have more prominent inattentive features of the disorder (predominantly inattentive presentation), while another may be more impulsive or hyperactive (predominantly hyperactive presentation), and a third family member may have symptoms related to all domains (combined presentation). This can even be true when the disorder is present in identical twins. Within a family, girls with ADHD are more frequently identified as "inattentive" whereas boys with ADHD are more frequently identified as "hyperactive." In addition, the most prominent traits in a single individual may change over their lifetime or be more prominent in different environments. For example, a child whose main identified symptom in elementary school was difficulty sitting still and being disruptive may grow into an adult whose only significant symptom is difficulty paying attention during business meetings. This is why all the various presentations are lumped together as "ADHD." As stated in Chapter 1, what used to be called "ADD" is now considered a specific "presentation" of ADHD (that is, predominantly inattentive).

The reason why ADHD runs in families mostly has to do with **genes**. So do we know which genes are involved? Can we do a genetic test to see if someone has ADHD? The short answer, for now, is mostly "no," although that may change with time, as science is always progressing and improving. For the purposes of this book, there are a few general points worth making about the genetics of ADHD.

First, as with most behavioral conditions, the genetics of ADHD is extremely complex. There are several components to this complexity:

- There are many **loci** that confer risk for ADHD in the human **genome**. Current estimates are that small differences (or

variants) at around 7,000 loci (different spots in human DNA) account for about 90% of the genetics of ADHD.
- Each one of these variants has a small effect by itself. That is, most people with ADHD do not have it because of a single variant, but because of combined small effects from having a large number of variants acting together.
- Different people with ADHD have different variants. In one person with ADHD, the principal variants responsible may be "A," "R," "X," and "Z." In another person with ADHD, the responsible variants may instead be "B," "D," "I," "V," and "W."
- The same variants that are associated with ADHD also contribute to other psychiatric disorders. Even though psychiatric illnesses such as major depression, schizophrenia, bipolar disorder, and ADHD seem very different in terms of their symptoms, the underlying genetics overlap heavily.
- The effect of most variants is only partly expressive and penetrant. This means that even if two people happen to have the same variants (that is, identical twins), one might have ADHD while the other might have a different psychiatric condition such as autism or schizophrenia—or even no psychiatric condition at all.

If you think through these five points, you will understand why scientists have not yet identified all the genes involved in ADHD, and also why you can't just go and get a genetic test to tell you whether or not you have the disorder. For starters, you could have a lot of variants associated with ADHD and still not have the disorder. Therefore, even though we know genetics plays an important role in ADHD, there is no way (at present) to do a genetic test to determine if you do or do not have ADHD.

Is ADHD Partly a Matter of Chance?

Chance *does* play a role in whether someone has ADHD. We will probably never get to the point where we can predict with 100%

certainty who has or will develop this or that medical or neuropsychiatric condition, because an element of chance is always involved, including during brain development both before and after birth. Even if you had complete and accurate knowledge of someone's genetic risk for ADHD and also knew precisely how to combine that information with all their other risk factors (for example, socioeconomic status, exposure to stress, exposure to environmental toxins), you still couldn't predict the outcome for sure.

That is why two people with identical genes (that is, identical twins), even though they resemble each other more than two average siblings do, still don't have identical personalities, let alone identical neuropsychiatric conditions. If twin #1 has had tough experiences, a few "bad breaks" in life, or even just some bad luck while their brain was developing in utero, while twin #2 had more positive experiences overall, twin #1 might develop a mental health problem while twin #2 might not.

Summary: Implications of Biology for ADHD Diagnosis and Treatment

To summarize, in this chapter we sought to give you state-of-the-art information around the biological sciences connected to ADHD. We realize a lot of it was technical and may be overdetailed. We hope to leave you with just a few major takeaway points relevant to your journey as someone with ADHD or as someone who loves and cares for somebody else with ADHD.

ADHD must necessarily arise from differences in the structure and activity of the brain, but current science has not firmly identified what those differences are in a way that facilitates diagnosis or treatment. The main reason for this is that many brain structures and circuits are involved, and the changes and differences among them are extremely small and overlap with normal variation. Similarly, ADHD runs in families and so we know that genes are involved, but the relevant genetic differences are so many and so small and have such variable effects that there is no genetic test that can reliably identify people with ADHD or reliably tell you what medications will work best for you or your loved one with ADHD. One day, this will come, possibly even sooner than we might imagine—but for now it remains science fiction.

CHAPTER 4

What Causes ADHD?

Society and Environment

In this chapter, you will learn:

- How the environment and culture contribute to ADHD
- About ADHD in marginalized communities
- About contributions from other mental health challenges (comorbidity)

In Chapter 3, we discussed the biological basis for ADHD. But as with every neuropsychiatric condition—indeed, as with every medical condition—causation is not just about anatomy or genes; it's also about contributions from the environment and culture. This chapter is dedicated to these other important factors that may cause or worsen ADHD.

Contributions of the Environment and Culture to ADHD

The type of science that studies these factors in medicine is called **epidemiology**. Epidemiological studies have identified environmental factors that influence ADHD. Moreover, some studies have distinguished environmental factors that appear to affect people with ADHD differently depending on their sex or that might primarily impact the development of inattentive versus hyperactive symptom domains of ADHD.

It is important to note that, in general, epidemiological evidence tends to be correlational rather than **causal**. This means that a study may be able to show that ADHD and some other factor might both be present at the same time, but that doesn't necessarily prove the factor *caused* ADHD. One limitation is that epidemiological studies are often retrospective. An example of a retrospective study is one in which researchers ask mothers of children diagnosed with ADHD what they did years ago while pregnant, or search medical or other records to collect this information after the fact. This type of research depends on the accuracy and completeness of the medical record, or (more questionably) on a person remembering and accurately reporting their former behavior.

One of the strongest correlations in ADHD is **bioenvironmental**. While environmental factors are sometimes implicated in ADHD, and biological factors (see Chapter 3) are as well, the strongest correlation is actually between the environment and the biology of a given person with ADHD, both of which then contribute to the likelihood of developing ADHD.

For example, if the use of nicotine during pregnancy correlates with the development of ADHD in the child, is that because nicotine exposure during pregnancy affects the child's brain development in a way that leads directly to ADHD? That could be true, but there are other possibilities. There could be genetic factors shared by the mother and baby that contribute to an increased risk of nicotine addiction in the mother and that separately contribute to increased risk of ADHD in her baby. Alternatively, the fact that the mother smokes could be a reaction to living in a psychologically stressful environment, and it could be the stressful environment, rather than the smoking, that contributes to the development of ADHD in the child. In fact, it is likely that the correlation we observe between a mother smoking and her child having ADHD is a result of all these factors working together. Similarly, if an epidemiological study finds that poverty correlates with ADHD, is that because ADHD causes poverty, or because poverty causes ADHD? Perhaps both are true: ADHD could lead people to have less financial success; that could in turn lead to increased stress, and that could then worsen ADHD symptoms in an individual or contribute to it in their children—a vicious cycle. With these caveats in mind, here is what we know:

Drug Use

There is a substantial correlation between ADHD and substance use problems. As stated in the above example, does this mean that drug use contributes to the development of ADHD, or that ADHD leads to an increased risk for drug use? Again, perhaps both are true. Either way, there is a strong correlation between these factors across the life cycle.

Prenatal Drug Exposure

Some studies say that yes, smoking cigarettes, drinking alcohol, or using illicit drugs such as heroin can increase an individual's likelihood of having a child with ADHD; other studies say no. The truth is that although there is some reason to be suspicious, there is no hard-and-fast research proving that mild or modest drug use during pregnancy causes ADHD. That said, higher levels of drug use do tend to correlate with greater concern for any adverse birth outcome (including ADHD)—but, again, very little can be pointed to in terms of a proof of direct causation.

Postnatal Drug Use

There is a theory that people with ADHD gravitate toward substance use to relieve ADHD symptoms; this is commonly known as "self-medication." There is also some evidence that people with ADHD are slightly more prone to become physiologically addicted to certain substances compared to the general population. Among the most common drugs of addiction—caffeine, nicotine, cocaine, and methamphetamine—affect the brain in somewhat similar ways to the prescription stimulant medications used to treat ADHD. However, there are important differences that make these substances less effective for managing ADHD symptoms and also more addicting than ADHD medications. (Yes, you read that correctly: Caffeine and nicotine are more addictive than stimulant medications when used as prescribed.) **THC**, the most psychoactive component in **cannabis**, may have some positive effects on impulsivity and distractibility, but it is not helpful for many other aspects of attention, and over time it tends to worsen motivation—clearly, this is not therapeutic for anyone struggling with ADHD. Other commonly abused drugs, such as alcohol or opiates, have no conceivable therapeutic benefit in ADHD.

In general, use of non-prescription **psychoactive drugs** adversely impacts reliable performance and creates or exacerbates rather than alleviates most cognitive challenges. For someone with ADHD who is struggling at baseline with these issues, concurrent drug use can only make things worse over time, as well as make their symptoms more difficult to tease apart, diagnose, and treat correctly. So even if a person with ADHD initially turns to a drug to compensate for their ADHD symptoms, most people with ADHD who also abuse substances wind up doing so to psychologically escape from the negative consequences of their ADHD—rather than to treat it.

Psychological Stress

In recent years, more and more studies have correlated psychological stress at all stages of the life cycle with the prevalence of ADHD.

Prenatal Exposure

Maternal psychological stress is a potential contributing factor for many neuropsychiatric disorders, including ADHD. Studies are fairly consistent in showing that many types of psychological stress during pregnancy (for example, stress arising from the death of a loved one) can influence the later development of ADHD in the child. We don't really know how that works or exactly how much stress can be tolerated before it begins to have negative effects or how reversible those effects may be. It likely depends on the individual personality of the mother, as well as the baby's genetic susceptibility to stress.

Stress During Infancy

At least a few studies have shown that psychological stress during infancy and the toddler years may be a risk factor for ADHD. Examples of this type of stress may include being in foster care or an orphanage or witnessing violent interpersonal exchanges or events. Once again, there is the problem of separating correlation from causation: Violent interpersonal exchanges and events are more likely to occur in a household in which one or both parents have ADHD. So if children from such a household are more likely to develop ADHD, is that because of the events the children witnessed or because they inherited ADHD from their parents? As usual, we are left saying both could be true.

During Childhood and Adolescence

In the late 1990s, some studies suggested that factors such as poverty or growing up with family conflict (which could include an absent parent or a parent with a psychiatric disorder) could contribute to ADHD, especially in boys, and that these issues persisted long after the children grew up and left their childhood homes. It's really hard to do these studies well and also difficult to know what aspects of poverty or family conflict are most important to consider. For example, it could be that poor nutrition as a result of poverty is the critical link, or perhaps being in a less stable social situation, or experiencing a lack of opportunities to develop skills, or once again it could be that the parents in these households are more likely to have ADHD themselves and then pass it on genetically to their children. Most likely it is some combination of all of the above.

Toxins

Lead exposure, which in the United States has historically come from children ingesting flakes of paint containing lead that had fallen off the walls of old homes, has been associated with ADHD in numerous studies. Other **heavy metals**, such as **mercury** and **arsenic**, are also neurotoxins associated with ADHD. Studies from different populations around the world have shown an increase in ADHD, along with some other neurodevelopmental conditions such as autism, in areas where these substances have polluted food or water sources.

Sugar, Artificial Ingredients, and Artificial Colors

Since about the mid-1970s, sugar has been widely considered to be a cause of hyperactivity. To this day, many people associate sugar intake with hyperactivity, but this association is actually based on very little scientific evidence. For example, many parents observe that their kids become **hyperkinetic** at events involving the consumption of large amounts of sugar (such as at a birthday party), but the connection between sugar intake and this hyperactivity is unclear. Maybe the child's excitement is from all the other forms of stimulation at the party, or from the color additives in the cake.

In the 1970s, Dr. Benjamin Feingold proposed that children who were allergic to aspirin might also react poorly to chemicals related to aspirin, including many artificial food dyes. He proposed a diet that removed artificial dyes, food preservatives, and artificial sweeteners as a treatment for hyperactivity and other behavioral disorders in children. The "Feingold Diet" caught on for a while, but it's very difficult to follow and its results for treating ADHD remain inconclusive.

It's fair to say that for most people with ADHD, a diet free of artificial ingredients does not seem to significantly improve their symptoms. **Elimination diets** are regimens where foodstuffs thought to worsen ADHD are eliminated from the diet, generally in children (no significant studies have been done in adults). For example, children will spend a few weeks eating nothing but a few different foods, and their ADHD symptoms are rated before and after. A major problem with interpreting any study involving elimination diets is that the children participating in the study invariably have highly motivated parents who are already primed to believe that diet impacts their child's behavior. In other words, these studies are biased in terms of participant selection, and as such are difficult to interpret. The bottom line is that while a person with ADHD might see a positive effect when eliminating artificial coloring and sweeteners from their diet, effects are typically small and such diets require a tremendous amount of discipline to achieve if you're an adult with ADHD or to enforce for your child if you're a parent. In our opinion, putting yourself or a loved one on a special diet in the hopes of improving ADHD symptoms is likely more trouble than it's worth for most people.

Dietary Supplements

Dietary supplementation with omega-3 fatty acids, found in fish, walnuts, and flax and chia seeds - or with saffron, have been found to have statistically significant positive effects on ADHD symptoms in some studies. It must be emphasized that for most patients the effect of such dietary supplementation is negligible compared to the benefits from taking a prescription medication, and there may be side effects as well. This gap in effectiveness is even more substantial when it comes to mineral supplementation. While a few unreplicated studies have reported correlations between ADHD and low levels of certain dietary minerals such as iron, copper, and zinc, no study has ever shown that supplementation with these minerals significantly improves symptoms of ADHD.

Electronic Distractions/Diversions

Smartphones, tablets, and other electronic devices have become a major influence on our lives. Children now get started on them as toddlers and children, when they are in a position to affect brain development. The full effect this has on brain development is still unknown and is a matter for research to decipher. But even without doing research, everyone implicitly understands that doing anything for hours each day is bound to influence how your mind works. And there is already evidence, from **electroencephalograms** (EEGs) and sophisticated brain imaging, that using electronic devices for multiple hours a day affects both your brain's activity and how it is wired.

Does the use of these devices increase the risk of ADHD? Nobody can say for sure yet, and it is likely that the answer depends on the specific device and what it is being used for. For example, solo videogames that emphasize continuous action or violence are more likely to affect attention negatively when compared to games that require complex problem solving or that are part of a shared social experience. That said, as the use of screens has increased in our society, our attention span has been steadily decreasing. For example, research has shown that in 2003, people could be attentive to a screen for an average of 2½ minutes. By 2012, that time went down to 75 seconds, and in the last few years, it diminished further to just 47 seconds. This correlates with changes in how media are presented. In films and TV, directors are changing shots faster than they used to. In 1930, the average shot length was 12 seconds. Now, it's not uncommon for movie shots to change every 4 seconds or even faster. Shot length for the *Iron Man* and *Bourne* movie series, for example, decreased from an average of 3.5 seconds in the first movie to closer to 2 seconds by the third movie. And many young people today program their phones to routinely deliver YouTube, Instagram, or similar video content at double the "normal" speed.

There are electronic devices and videogames that have recently been cleared by the U.S. Food and Drug Administration (FDA) to improve ADHD. That said, with few exceptions, the electronic devices and media we use every day have attributes that are unlikely to promote attention, decrease impulsivity, and improve other aspects of ADHD—and many seem more likely to do the opposite.

When we watch TV or scroll Instagram, we are experiencing something passively, without having to think very much. As we watch our shows or scroll through social media, we are seeing something very artificial, but are generally unconscious of the scripts, makeup, lighting, and added sound effects used in the making of the video. The worlds shown in these media are carefully constructed to be easy and relatable. When we lift our eyes and look at the real world, we see people who don't look so perky, houses that don't look so neat and stylish, and dialogue that is not so quick and snappy. The real world becomes less attractive and harder to pay attention to compared to this made-up world. When someone who is used to electronic devices, videogames, and social media says "I'm bored," it often means "my real world is not as exciting, fun, or easy to digest as my device's world."

The use of devices also makes us less able to persist in the face of difficulties. On a device, if you like something, you stick with it, but if you don't, you can just swipe it away. The real world is not like that. In real life, we have to know how to face challenging situations without avoiding them. We have to deal with people we don't like (or who don't like us), problems that challenge and stretch our personal comfort zones, or issues that take a long time to resolve. If you are on a device many hours per day and deal with uncomfortable things by swiping them away, you may get frustrated by your inability to do so in the real world.

How many hours spent per day on these devices is OK? No one really knows. It probably depends on the individual as well as what they are doing on the devices. As a general rule, we recommend not being on a device longer than the time you spend on your real-world hobbies. You (or your child) should not be on a device longer than the time you spend on activities like reading, playing an instrument, gardening, doing sports, or playing board games. It's important that a child or adult can find a way to develop interests at a real-world level, as such activities require building attention, controlling impulses, and mastering body movements—all challenges for someone with ADHD. Electronic devices, by presenting an "easy" and manufactured world that requires little of this from the user, make it that much harder to build these skills.

> Seventeen-year-old Savannah was a junior in high school. She came for an evaluation because she saw a TikTok video about ADHD that reminded her of herself "and anyway, my friends all think I have ADHD." During the evaluation, it became evident that the features and behaviors she noticed had started squarely in seventh grade, when she got her first phone. Before that, Savannah had been attentive and responsible. In the seventh grade she started to miss many assignments. She would often start her homework around midnight and then had to get up at 7:30 a.m. to go to school. She often complained she didn't have time or energy to do her homework earlier due to being in afterschool sports. However, she managed to squeeze in nearly 7 hours of social media scrolling per day (that is, nearly the equivalent of a full-time job).
>
> She felt that her phone was not the issue "because I put it away when I do homework and I still can't concentrate." We reviewed with her that her brain was constantly being "revved up" by her phone and that even when she put it down that effect was still present. Furthermore, Savannah was always tired due to a lack of adequate sleep, making it even harder for her to concentrate. In fact, she did start to feel (and perform) much better once she significantly cut down her daily phone use.

"Crazy Busy" Lives

In recent years, the term "crazy busy" has crept into common use, and with good reason: The world is moving faster and faster all the time. It's fair to ask whether this trend contributes to ADHD.

Starting with the age of electricity and more powerful electrical lighting, we have increased the number of productive hours in the day and have crammed more into each hour. Most children grow up in households where both parents are working, or else in a one-parent household with a full-time working parent. Parents are stretched thin, managing both the household chores and working for their livelihood. Work is often high pressure and involves responding to multiple inputs at once from phones, instant messages, emails, and meetings. There is less time for relaxation and hobbies, or for vacation, which is often the only time when people are not multitasking. In between (and often during) scheduled activities, we text, email, scroll, respond to notifications, and divert our attention from the task at hand. We are overscheduled and under-rested. There are many demands on our time, and we can easily overfill our days.

Think about the simple act of getting to work. People used to have just a few clothes, so deciding what to wear required hardly any attention. There were also few choices for breakfast. One parent might get the kids to school (kids having similarly few choices about what to wear or eat), while the other parent might go to work. Getting to work may have involved just walking out to the fields as a farmer, or walking or possibly riding a horse to town over a half-hour away, with nothing to do on the way but gaze at the nature around them. Nowadays our attention is diffused, as each person in the family has to choose what to wear and eat. There is often chaos (including that generated by electronic distractions) as everybody is getting up and out the door. The ride to work (or school) may be done at 60 mph, with scenery zipping by the window, and our cars often have multiple gauges, music, onboard computers, and phones dinging next to us the whole way.

No matter how your attention starts out, interrupting it to switch tasks due to over-crammed schedules and demands wears down your attention span. If you are used to having to change activities frequently throughout the day (for example, writing a response to an email and then getting interrupted by an IM or phone call), then you get in the habit of switching your attention frequently as well. Some of us have to respond to dozens (or even hundreds) of emails per day.

Switching tasks takes time for your brain to do. Dr. Gloria Mark, a psychologist and professor at University of California at Irvine, likens attention for a task to having a whiteboard in your mind. If you change tasks, the information on the whiteboard has to be erased and rewritten. That takes time. Sometimes your brain can't erase it completely, so you are still thinking about one task while starting on another. That leads to a lot of internal distractions, and also makes confusion more likely to occur in whatever task you are trying to do.

This creates a situation where we always feel behind. We always feel too busy. We must pay attention to so many things that our brains become exhausted. It becomes difficult to give anything more than brief and superficial focus. Instead of focusing, our brains keep expecting the next interruption. We become so revved up that it can be hard to adjust even when our schedule does calm down. When we finally have the opportunity to relax, it may take days to reduce the pace of our mind to a point where we can finally pay sustained and deep attention to just one thing at a time.

> *Forty-seven-year-old Maria was, by any standard, a busy woman. A working mother of three school-aged kids, she was constantly on the go. Her husband had a demanding job and was not as involved in the running of the household as she was—although her job was similarly demanding. She got up at 5:30 to go work out—or, as she called it, to have her "me time!" When she returned from the gym, she made sure the kids were dressed and fed, added needed food items to the shopping list, and drove two of the kids to school while her husband dropped the other one off.*

During the drive, texts flashed up on her onboard monitor. Maria worked as a sales rep—which involved constant checking of emails and answering of texts and phone calls, as well as somehow seeing her clients. She tended to procrastinate on completing her expense reports and documentation until the last second, and her boss was getting irritated at her lack of preparation for meetings. She tried to work as quickly as she could so she would be available to get her children to their various sports practices, music lessons, and playdates. She felt guilty if she had to say "no" to them and would smile and say, "We'll find a way to make it work."

Maria tried to cook dinner at least three nights per week, which also meant managing the grocery runs. She was also in charge of scheduling get-togethers with other couples for dinner or drinks. Although her husband did the dishes and repairs around the house, she managed the laundry and oversaw the kids' schedules and needs. If there was a doctor's visit to take them to, she did it. She also took the dogs to the groomers, went to the bank, and paid the bills. She and her husband finally collapsed into bed around 10:30 or 11 each night.

She felt bad because she forgot things sometimes: forgot to sign field trip slips, forgot where her kids' cleats went, and— oops!—forgot basketball practice one day. She scheduled a vacation and her daughter's birthday party for the same weekend. She would walk into a room to do something, get distracted by seeing the 10 other things she had to do and would forget why she came into the room in the first place. She often made silly mistakes at work.

She came in for an evaluation to report: "I feel like I'm losing it. I must have ADHD." The doctor told her that she did not have ADHD, but that the more things a person has on their plate, the harder it is for them to pay attention to any one thing. Maria solved her "ADHD" by not trying to be everything to everyone.

> She demanded more accountability and responsibility from her kids to manage their own belongings. She asked her husband to help more—which he was happy to do; he just didn't realize she needed the help. And because she was often distracted by her own thoughts of things she needed to do, she discovered it was helpful to keep a to-do list. Offloading these items to a piece of paper kept them out of her mind.

Exactly how much the recent increase in the rate of ADHD diagnosis is due to the increase in the rate and complexity of our lives is controversial. Some say that the increases in ADHD symptoms and diagnosis are simply a response to our "crazy busy" lives. But to the extent ADHD has been looked at rigorously, it appears people throughout history have had it, even though it wasn't called "ADHD" or considered a medical condition until the last few decades. While there is a popular notion that ADHD might have been helpful for people in certain roles in ancient times (that is, for "hunters" vs. "farmers"), this idea has not found much support in scientific studies. For example, **paleogenetics** has been used to trace risk variants for ADHD in the DNA of humans back to prehistoric times—back to when our ancestors were working with nothing but stone tools. The results suggest that as far back as scientists can look, the variants associated with ADHD have been selected against during human evolution. The bottom line is that, whether you believe it's sometimes helpful or not, humans have struggled with the challenges of ADHD for as long as they've been around. That said, it also stands to reason that the more things you have on your plate and the faster the world goes around, the more you will forget about some of the tasks you have to do, the more you will rush around and make mistakes, and the more you will feel unfocused, overwhelmed, and even paralyzed over where to begin a task. The modern situation of being "crazy busy" is challenging for everybody whether they have ADHD or not, and it is bound to make ADHD more challenging for those who do have it.

ADHD in Marginalized Communities

When it comes to examining the contributions of environment and culture to ADHD, marginalized communities are a special case. People who live in marginalized communities are likely to be at greater risk for developing ADHD because of the environmental pressures they live under, including all the aforementioned stressors. But at the same time, people who have ADHD and are part of this demographic are more likely to go undiagnosed.

The reasons for underdiagnosis in these communities is multifactorial. There is typically a relative lack of medical and mental health care professionals serving these communities. This compounds the fact that individuals within these communities have to spend more time and energy fulfilling day-to-day survival priorities and have correspondingly less time and energy to consider seeking diagnosis and treatment for any attentional or other mental health problems. Some people in these communities have not had prior positive experiences with doctors or may belong to groups with a history of maltreatment by professionals, and may harbor fears of being labeled and further marginalized by a diagnosis as a result. Among immigrant groups, there may be increased stigma and reticence around mental illness treatment related to their culture of origin. Individuals within these groups sometimes have been exposed to more misinformation than people in other groups. They may be sensitized to being controlled by other groups and may correspondingly be more concerned about issues such as a fear of "mind control." As a result of these and other factors, individuals with ADHD from marginalized groups are more likely to go undiagnosed or to be misdiagnosed with other mental health problems such as oppositional defiant disorder or conduct disorder.

Contributions from Other Mental Health Challenges

Many psychiatric conditions tend to be **comorbid**: that is, two or more conditions often occur together in the same patient. ADHD is highly comorbid with other mental health, as well as general health, conditions. In some cases, a person doesn't have ADHD at all, but instead has other conditions that are actually fully responsible for the symptoms they are experiencing. In some other individuals, ADHD is a big part of their problem, even if it's not their only problem.

Exact estimates vary widely, but it is fair to say that compared to the general population, adults with ADHD are anywhere from two to 10 times more likely to have a mood disorder such as major depression, an anxiety disorder such as generalized anxiety, or a substance use disorder such as **alcoholism**. The converse is also true: People with major depression are far more likely to have ADHD, and the same goes for anxiety disorders and substance abuse. In some studies, as many as 40% of the participants who had depression, anxiety, or a substance use problem also had ADHD.

> *Jeremy, age 26, had difficulty keeping jobs and became convinced that each time he started a new one, it was only a matter of time before he'd get fired. Over time, he bothered less and less to even try to succeed with each new position. But this also caused him to become self-conscious and anxious when he did have a job and depressed and hopeless when he didn't.*
>
> *Eventually, Jeremy withdrew socially, both because he didn't enjoy being around people who were successful and happy and also because he was convinced people didn't really want to be around him. Jeremy began spending more and more of his time playing videogames and smothering his sorrows in daily alcohol and cannabis use.*

> Only after his parents intervened and took him to a professional for help was he diagnosed with major depression, generalized anxiety disorder, and also alcohol and cannabis abuse. But it took another few years before an astute clinician finally questioned Jeremy about the attentional problems that got him into trouble in the first place and suggested the possibility that Jeremy should also be diagnosed with and treated for ADHD.

The signs and symptoms of ADHD can often be masked, which is why it is so important to answer your physician's questions honestly and not to be embarrassed to share what's going on in your life. Some of the questions asked by your provider may sound personal, and you may not want to share the information. You may not want to share how many hours you spend scrolling on your phone or details about your intake of drugs or alcohol. But it is always important that your doctor, therapist, or nurse practitioner understand the "whole picture." A patient may come to a doctor asking for help for the one issue they feel is important to address, but may actually have highly intertwined problems in multiple areas. In general, issues resulting from ADHD tend to be interwoven with other issues, and these problems "feed off" one another. So, addressing just one problem (such as ADHD) while ignoring other aspects of a person's emotional and behavioral landscape (for example, anxiety levels, mood, amount of sleep, or substance use) is seldom successful.

Sometimes depression or anxiety is the most obvious aspect of a patient's poor functioning, and the doctor may therefore focus on those. However, if treatment for the depression and anxiety is not working well enough, they may want to raise the possibility of ADHD, as the symptoms can be very similar. When treatment for depression or anxiety fails to improve symptoms, adding a treatment for ADHD may be the key.

On a positive note, because ADHD can be interwoven into so many aspects of your life, if you can give your doctor all the information, treating one condition will often improve the others as well. For example, if your ADHD is treated, your sleep, anxiety, and mood may improve as well. If you are the parent of a child with ADHD, you may be relieved to see your child worry less and believe in themselves more once they start an effective treatment plan.

We hope this perspective will help you be honest with your doctor, even with the embarrassing questions. We also hope your provider will use the information you give them compassionately, rather than judgmentally. We discuss the overlap between ADHD and other psychiatric and medical conditions more fully in the next chapter.

CHAPTER 5

Could My ADHD Actually Be Something Else?

In this chapter, you will learn:

- How other factors can mimic or worsen ADHD
- How conditions such as depression, anxiety, bipolar disorder, obsessive–compulsive disorder, psychosis, autism spectrum disorder, and dementia can mimic ADHD
- How substance use and addiction can mimic ADHD
- How poor sleep can mimic ADHD
- How medical conditions such as obstructive sleep apnea and absence seizures can mimic ADHD

How Other Factors Can Mimic or Worsen ADHD

ADHD is basically a disorder in which people have trouble regulating certain types of behavior. Specifically, a person with ADHD has trouble regulating their attention, and (in some people) also their impulses, movement, and perhaps even emotional reactions. But there are other reasons why people can experience these same types of behavioral challenges. This is important because other conditions that cause similar challenges may have very different solutions, including different medical, psychological, and behavioral treatments. If these other causes aren't addressed, treating "ADHD" will not necessarily improve the situation, no matter which ADHD medications are tried or how much ADHD coaching is received.

Another important point is that the answer to whether a person has ADHD or something else is not always an "either/or" determination—in fact, it rarely is. A person may have poor focus or impulse control because of ADHD, but these challenges may also be worsened by other conditions, either all the time or some of the time. If that is the case, until these other conditions are addressed, the ADHD will never be well controlled. You or your loved one may incorrectly think a different type of ADHD treatment is needed, when really some other issue needs to be addressed. In these situations, the ADHD medication (Chapter 6) or coaching or therapy (Chapter 7) is still working. The problem is that an ADHD treatment has to have something to work with: the ADHDer's brain. If the brain isn't working optimally for some other reason, the ADHD treatment may not help until that problem is addressed.

Psychiatric Conditions

Other psychiatric conditions often adversely affect the way the brain processes information—including the ability to focus, think clearly and logically, feel motivated, and organize tasks. In some cases, such symptoms can closely mimic ADHD. Major depression, generalized anxiety disorder, and even bipolar disorder are often mistaken for ADHD. Conversely, untreated ADHD can be (and often is) mistaken for these other conditions. We use the term **diagnostic mimicry** to describe this phenomenon. It can take a very skilled and experienced clinician to tell the difference between ADHD and another condition that causes similar or overlapping symptoms.

It is not uncommon for a person who has depression or anxiety to notice a degradation in their memory or in their ability to think as the first sign they are having a problem. It can sometimes be challenging for a doctor to convince a patient that what they really need is treatment for depression or anxiety, as opposed to a brain scan or a stimulant medication.

Charlie is a 32-year-old lawyer who, with the benefit of hindsight, now realizes he has struggled with ADHD all his life, but who only got diagnosed and started treatment for it 2 years ago. At the time of his diagnosis, he was seeking help because of problems both at work and at home. His psychiatrist prescribed a stimulant medication that, after some initial dose adjustments, did wonders for him, literally transforming his life. It helped him stay focused and organized, helped him manage his many tasks and obligations both at work and at home, and greatly improved interactions with his wife. It had been working well and consistently for him until about 2 months ago.

He makes an appointment to see his psychiatrist and tells him that for the past 2 months, his ADHD medication has stopped working. When he's taken it lately, it doesn't seem to do anything. He asks if the dose should be increased, or if he should try a completely different pill, and states he favors the latter option. Upon further discussion, he admits he has already tried taking an extra dose of the medicine a few times on his own, but it didn't seem to help. Taking the extra medicine just made him feel jittery and even a little physically ill and panicky, something he had never experienced when taking it before.

The doctor agrees to consider a medication switch, and then asks Charlie what else has been going on in his life. Charlie states that he and his wife have been fighting more lately. She complains he has been ignoring their relationship in favor of his career, which he admits has been a lot more stressful lately. A few months ago, he got a promotion, and that has meant additional responsibilities and assignments. His sleep has been poor; he finds himself ruminating about tasks he needs to complete at work and minor daily aggravations, both at bedtime and when he wakes up in the middle of the night. Frequently, he is awake for an hour or more before he finally manages to fall back asleep and has trouble getting up in the morning. He's

> stopped exercising regularly, but even so, his weight is down because he doesn't have much of an appetite. He had to push himself to go to a pro basketball game last weekend—and he only briefly enjoyed being at the game even though he was there with some old buddies, they had great seats, and their team won.
>
> His psychiatrist diagnoses Charlie with depression and prescribes him an antidepressant that he says will also improve his sleep and reduce his anxiety. Charlie is skeptical about taking another type of medication—after all, it took him almost 30 years to accept his ADHD diagnosis and take a pill for that. But he's grown to trust this doctor, and so he agrees to give it a try.
>
> A few weeks after starting the antidepressant medication, Charlie is feeling somewhat better. His sleep is still not 100% back to normal but it has improved, and he is ruminating less. His appetite is also improved, and he finds himself laughing again—he hadn't even realized that was missing until after it came back. He and his wife still have significant issues, and he remains concerned about their future together, but they're talking again, and they've decided to see a relationship counselor together. One of the most remarkable things to Charlie is that his ADHD medication has started working again and at exactly the same dose it always worked at before.

In general, it is very unusual for ADHD medications to suddenly stop working. If they worked for your ADHD once, they will generally keep working (though sometimes the dose may need a little adjusting, especially in the first few months of treatment). If your longstanding ADHD medication has seemed to stop working recently, your doctor will likely look for some other cause for the problem. Frequently, the explanation is that some other factor is adversely impacting your ability to pay attention or control your impulses. This could be a major depressive episode or generalized anxiety, but it could also be one of many other types of psychiatric conditions, and it is often difficult to tease them apart.

> *Forty-year-old Samir has been treated on and off for ADHD for the past 15 years. He is back to see his provider because he feels his "mind is racing." This happens at work, where his performance reviews are lackluster, but also in the evenings as he is trying to fall asleep. Upon interview he seems happy, is very personable, talks a bit fast, and flits from topic to topic very conversationally—but he is also fully cooperative and answers all questions put to him by his doctor.*

In this and the next two examples, you will notice some ambiguity about what is causing the patient's problems. It is possible that Samir's ADHD is at the root of at least some of what is going on with him, but he could also be hypomanic or manic. Can we attribute his subjectively racing mind, lack of sleep, and rapidly shifting, highly conversational speech to baseline ADHD combined with recent stress? Or do these symptoms reflect some other psychiatric problem, like bipolar disorder?

> *Joanna, a 28-year-old woman, has never sought psychiatric or psychological help, despite some longstanding issues with procrastination. When she was young and living with her parents, they helped keep her on task and on time; later on, the structure of her job was very helpful. But now she finds herself juggling a husband, a toddler, being a homemaker, and trying to manage a job, all at once. She has so much to do she can't possibly stay on top of it all. She looks around at all the things that require her attention, pulling her in different directions, and feels completely overwhelmed. She doesn't even know where to begin! She reports that the other day, for the first time in her life, she may have had a panic attack.*

Joanna is very anxious. Does she have panic disorder and need treatment for that? Or will a stimulant for ADHD help get her thoughts and tasks organized, reduce her procrastination, get her to be more productive, and therefore make her feel calmer and more in control of her life? Maybe both are true.

> *After his father, who had ADHD, died in a car accident, 15-year-old Lewis seemed to do OK for about a year, but then his grades started to slip. His mother notes that middle school was easy for him—he never had to study to get A's on tests. Now, in high school, his grades are dropping to C's and D's, and he seems increasingly unmotivated and even listless. A month ago, for the first time ever, he didn't complete some required assignments for class, and his teachers contacted his mother out of concern. For the past few weeks, he hasn't been sleeping well; he told his mother that last night, an argument coming from next door kept him up most of the night. He lives in a free-standing home, and his mother heard nothing unusual.*

Lewis lost his father last year, and he may now be depressed: That would explain his lackluster academic performance and poor sleep, and could even lead to him hearing voices. But he is also at an age when primary psychotic disorders like schizophrenia first arise, and the onset of an illness like that is also often precipitated by psychological stress. Is that why he is doing so poorly, seems listless, and heard voices in his bedroom last night? Then again, maybe Lewis has ADHD. It is hereditary, and his father had it; maybe the level of work he is expected to accomplish in high school has finally caught up with him. If he can't keep up in school anymore, that would affect his self-esteem and motivation, and perhaps the neighbors next door really were yelling at each other last night and his mother slept through it all.

Hopefully Samir, Joanna, and Lewis all have good doctors with enough experience to carefully sort through the details and tell the difference between ADHD, bipolar disorder, panic disorder, and a psychotic break!

Depression

Depressed people often do not have the energy or motivation to start tasks or get things done. Tasks seem harder and procrastination is worse. The ability to concentrate and think clearly can be adversely affected, and, as mentioned above, for some depressed people this is actually the first symptom they notice. People who are depressed are also more likely to notice when things go wrong rather than when they go right and get discouraged more easily. All of this can look a lot like ADHD.

A list of potential symptoms and signs of depression adapted from the DSM-5 include:

- Pervasive depressed mood
- Difficulty finding interest or pleasure in many activities
- Significant weight loss or weight gain due to change in appetite
- Slowing of movements and thoughts
- Near-constant fatigue/poor energy
- Feeling guilty for no reason, feeling worthless
- Reduced ability to think or concentrate, or indecisiveness, nearly every day
- Having thoughts of death or suicide

Note that a diminished ability to think or concentrate is among the main symptoms and signs (#7) of depression. Cognitive slowing, symptom #4, can also be confused with inattentive ADHD. Depression and ADHD often coexist, so whether somebody is suffering from depression or ADHD is often not an "either/or" proposition. In fact, people with ADHD are far more likely to be depressed than people without ADHD.

Anxiety

People who are anxious also may have difficulty with paying attention. As we all know from personal experience, when you are very worried about something, it can be difficult to concentrate on anything else. See, for example, these signs of generalized anxiety disorder, adapted from the DSM-5:

- Excessive worry for at least 6 months
- Worry that is hard to control and that frequently shifts topics
- At least three of the following:
    - Edginess or restlessness
    - Feeling very tired/overwhelmed
    - Worse concentration; mind "blanking out"
    - Irritability
    - Aches and pains
    - Sleep difficulties

Once again, there is crossover between ADHD and this otherwise separate diagnosis. Symptoms and signs of generalized anxiety disorder include not only impaired concentration, which obviously can be mistaken for the inattentiveness of ADHD, but also edginess or restlessness, which can be confused with the fidgetiness of hyperactive ADHD. Moreover, just as with depression, there is a lot of **comorbidity**—many people who are anxious also have ADHD, and many people with ADHD are anxious, often as a result of feeling overwhelmed by all they need to do combined with their inability to focus, which makes it difficult to make progress on their to-do list.

How Anxiety and Depression Can Mimic ADHD

When it comes to the relationship between ADHD and either anxiety or depression, it can be hard to figure out whether a person's difficulties with concentration and focus are causing them to experience negative emotions or if the opposite is true. It's a "chicken-and-egg"

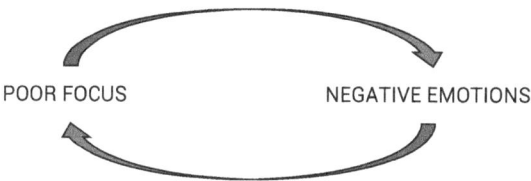

FIGURE 5.1 A feedback loop between poor focus and negative emotions creates a vicious cycle where both continually get worse.

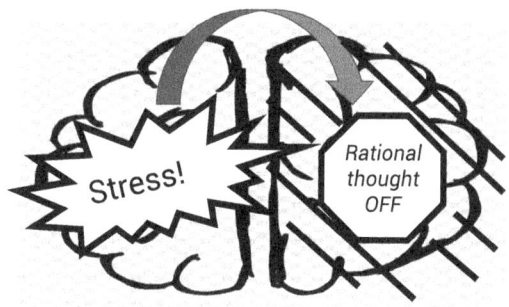

FIGURE 5.2 "Stressed" regions of your brain can turn off rational thinking regions.

problem, because these aspects of a person's mental life are linked together in another one of those "vicious cycles" we've discussed throughout this book. That is, a problem with one leads to a problem with the other; a feedback loop leads back from the second thing to the first thing again, and so on (Figure 5.1).

When someone has poor focus, it can lead to a lot of anxiety or sadness. But, when anxiety and sadness are present, they make it harder to focus. As a vast oversimplification, you can think of your brain as having two parts: the thinking/focus part and the emotional part. To simplify a lot of neuroanatomy, when the emotional part of your brain turns *on* due to negative emotions, that tends to turn *off* the thinking part of your brain. In other words, a person who is upset can't think properly. That's this particular biology in action (Figure 5.2).

The point is, sometimes it is hard to tell if a person is not concentrating because they are upset (that is, depressed or anxious) or because they have ADHD. And it could be both!

Bipolar Disorder

Bipolar disorder is most often diagnosed in adults but can be present in some children and can appear with ADHD-like symptoms in some cases. People with bipolar disorder appear very "moody." They have "down times" when they are depressed, which can look like ADHD or combine with ADHD in the same way depression does (see the section on depression above). But people with bipolar disorder can also have a mood swing that takes them in the opposite direction, called **mania** or (if less severe) **hypomania**. In this state, their mood is usually very good, even euphoric or grandiose—although they can also be irritable and impatient. People with hypomania or mania talk more rapidly and "tangentially"—that is, they flit quickly from one idea to the next, losing track of where they started. They may also be more distractible and impulsive, engage in more reward-seeking behavior, and have trouble sitting still. All of this can resemble ADHD, although there are important differences between ADHD and bipolar disorder that an experienced psychiatrist or psychologist should be able to distinguish.

Obsessive–Compulsive Disorder (OCD)

OCD is another condition that can create difficulties with focusing. OCD involves a pattern of unwanted thoughts (obsessions) that a person thinks about over and over again. They may also have compulsions—ritual behaviors they feel compelled to complete because not doing so causes anxiety. It is a bit less common for OCD to be diagnostically confused with ADHD, but it can sometimes cause a person to be unable to accomplish tasks. For example, if your child is obsessed with the number 3, it may be hard for them to complete math problems or write papers or read whenever the number 3 is involved (or perhaps if it is missing). To take another example, it may take a person with OCD much longer to complete their work because they obsessionally feel that they can't turn a page if they erased anything on it. Or, if they feel they have to do a ritual such as lining their pens or papers up in a certain way before getting started on a test, they may run out of time. The obsessions and compulsions in OCD are distressing—they are not things that people with OCD particularly want to think about or do, and so they often do not easily talk about them. In a child with OCD who doesn't easily talk about their obsessions and compulsions, the cause of their low accomplishment may be misattributed to poor concentration and be labeled inappropriately as ADHD. At the same time, comorbid ADHD can exacerbate OCD because the lack of focus from ADHD may make the person with OCD more doubtful about what they already did or thought. If you're already prone to obsessing and repeating and then, because of ADHD, think: "Wait, did I do that correctly? I wasn't paying close enough attention. I'm not sure," you're going to repeat that obsession or compulsion. In this way, comorbid ADHD in someone with OCD can exacerbate obsessions and compulsions.

Psychosis

Even the psychotic disorder schizophrenia has, as one of its central characteristics, difficulties with thinking that include cognitive slowing and problems with concentration and focus. This can sometimes be mistaken for ADHD in both the early stages of schizophrenia and later on as it progresses. In the early phases of schizophrenia, before a patient experiences any hallucinations or delusions, they may experience cognitive slowing, low motivation, or difficulties with thinking and paying attention. These issues are also among the most difficult aspects of schizophrenia to treat. Thus, a person with schizophrenia who has been successfully stabilized on medication and no longer has any hallucinations or delusions may still experience "residual" symptoms of poor motivation and difficulty thinking, including with attention and memory. These patients sometimes seek treatment for ADHD, although they really have something else.

Autism Spectrum Disorder (ASD)

On the basis of symptom categorization, there is overlap between ASD and ADHD. Although previous editions of the DSM stated that the diagnoses of ASD and ADHD were mutually exclusive, the DSM-5 allows for their comorbidity. It should come as no surprise, then, that the co-diagnosis of ADHD and ASD is growing, especially as around 50% of children who fit the DSM-5 diagnostic criteria for ASD also fit the DSM-5 diagnostic criteria for ADHD. Conversely, around 15% of children who fit the diagnostic criteria for ADHD also fit the diagnostic criteria for ASD.

What are the chief differences between ADHD and ASD? ADHD is, at its core, a problem with attention and controlling impulses. ASD is, at its core, related to abnormal social behavior and engagement. Individuals with severe ASD may not interact with other people at all and can be completely nonverbal.

So where is the symptom overlap? For starters, both disorders make people appear less engaged. Inattentive behavior in ADHD may cause affected children or adults to miss social cues, a symptom that can cause ADHD to resemble mild ASD. Kids with ADHD have a higher rate of rejection by their peers than kids who do not have ADHD—this can lead to them being more withdrawn, which can sometimes resemble the lack of social engagement typical of ASD. People with both disorders may have, or develop, problems with empathy, as well as with facial recognition of emotions. Impulsive behavior and deficits in planning (executive functioning) are common to both disorders. Both disorders can include problems with appropriate responses in conversations. The autistic person may not understand subtleties in communication, whereas the ADHDer may not be listening or may get distracted and go off topic. Cognitive rigidity can also be a problem in both disorders. For example, in autism one of the core features is difficulty with flexibility—that is, always having to have things in certain ways. But a similar symptom can also be present in ADHD: Due to losing things frequently, the ADHDer may become compulsive about where they put things and may get very upset if the items are moved. Both disorders are more often found in the presence of intellectual disability or more specific learning disabilities such as those related to language, reading (for example, dyslexia), or motor skills.

The two conditions have overlapping biology, including at the level of genetic susceptibility and brain imaging findings. But you don't need to be a research scientist to notice this overlap. It's not uncommon for a family to have one child with ASD and another with ADHD.

At a practical level, how concerned should you be about which is the correct diagnosis for you or your child? Should you worry about whether you or your child has been properly diagnosed with ADHD versus ASD? While it may help you frame your child's difficulties, remember that the important issue is to understand and treat the difficulties themselves, not the overall diagnosis. Treatment of either condition should be based on what the challenges really are.

If you or your child has a diagnosis of either ADHD or ASD, your focus should be on treating the actual behavioral challenges, as opposed to a diagnosis listed in a book or on a website. If your child has specific challenges with hyperactivity and impulsivity, then look for behavioral strategies, therapy, coaching, or medications to address that particular problem. If you are an adult with ADHD and the main challenge you face daily is with how you interact socially, then you should focus on therapy and coaching to address that challenge. Many of the therapeutic techniques used in each disorder are similar. For example, positive reinforcement of desired behaviors, achieving consistent quality sleep, engaging in regular exercise, and assembling appropriate educational support or accommodations are important strategies in addressing both disorders.

Finally, there is overlap in the medications used to treat these two disorders. While there are generally more specific medications that have been approved by the U.S. Food and Drug Administration (FDA) for ADHD than for ASD, with both disorders, medication management should focus on targeting symptom improvement. If the goal is to improve attention, regardless of whether the primary diagnosis is ADHD or ASD, an FDA-approved medication for treating attention issues (that is, for ADHD) is likely to be helpful. Conversely, there are some medications that have been approved by the FDA for impulsive behaviors, such as aggression, in ASD. Although less commonly used for the impulsiveness of ADHD, these medications may occasionally be useful in ADHD if severe impulse control issues are present.

Always remember that just because one treatment approach has worked for another person with the same diagnosis, it may or may not be what works best for you or your child. This even extends to what has been FDA approved; there are many reasons why a medication or treatment may not have been FDA approved that have nothing to do with its effectiveness, let alone whether it is best for a specific diagnosis or a specific individual. Treatment must always be based on what's in the best interest of the individual patient. Every person with ADHD and/or ASD is a unique individual with a unique brain, mind, and condition; no patient is a statistic (remember, all medical statistics apply to groups of people, not individuals), nor can a person ever be fully encapsulated by a diagnosis that comes down to a list of symptom criteria.

Dementia

As stated throughout this book, a recent feature of ADHD is the recognition that it is most often a lifelong condition. This creates a situation where, occasionally, someone is brought in for a diagnosis of

ADHD when it is pretty clear that something else, or at least something more complex, is going on.

> *Alex, age 72, is brought in by his partner, Susan, out of concern for his recent memory problems. Alex says he has been more forgetful lately, but when pressed, he doesn't have a lot to say by way of examples. At that point, Susan jumps in. She says that Alex has been losing his car keys more—most notably, last week they found them in the fridge, and the other day, they realized he'd left them in the car overnight. He also misplaces objects around the home, and he often can't remember the names of their neighbors. Susan complains that Alex often forgets what he was doing in the middle of doing it—he'll be in a room and not remember what he came in there for.*
>
> *Notably, Alex and Susan recently received a notice about their yearly tax filing stating that it was late and that they'd owe a penalty. Alex insisted he'd sent it in, but when they went through their papers, they found that he had only completed a portion of the paperwork, which was still on his desk. Susan insists that none of this is new, and that Alex has been this way for years. She gives examples of him forgetting their anniversary and their daughter's birthday for decades, and says he's always been a bit of a "pack rat"—their garage is impossible to get through because of all the junk he's collected over the years. However, when pressed, she admits it's been getting much worse lately.*

In this case, does Alex have ADHD or an illness that causes dementia, such as Alzheimer disease? Or does he have both? He clearly has some emerging and worsening memory problems, but it's not inconceivable that for years he managed with low-level attentional issues that simply never rose to the point of needing treatment. Perhaps it's the case that now, under the additional stress of an illness that causes dementia, the attention and memory issues have risen to the surface and become a point of concern. On the other hand, it seems likely that the main driver in this case is dementia of some kind that deserves therapeutic attention first. The diagnosis and treatment is probably best left to a specialist in **geriatric medicine**, who can address these concerns in tandem, especially in the context of any other medical problems Alex may be having.

Addiction

Other conditions that can trigger ADHD-like challenges, exacerbate existing ADHD, or be a consequence of ADHD are substance abuse and other addictions. While it is possible that the active ingredient in cannabis (THC) can actually help a bit with impulse control, both short- and long-term use of cannabis exacerbates ADHD challenges by contributing to poor motivation, poor task management, and worsening attention. Alcohol has no arguable benefit on any behavioral or cognitive aspects of ADHD, either acutely or over the long term, and it certainly exacerbates ADHD symptoms and their negative consequences. Addictions to electronic devices or videogames similarly do not lead to better task management in other areas of life, instead exacerbating the behavioral challenges of ADHD. Unfortunately for all concerned, these issues are often part of a vicious cycle of cause and effect that can be extremely challenging if not impossible to disentangle from ADHD. See Chapter 4 for additional discussion.

Poor Sleep

A fairly common condition that can reduce the ability to focus in both children and adults is poor sleep—either too few hours of sleep or poor-quality sleep. Sleep is absolutely essential to proper brain function—whether or not a person has ADHD, if their brain isn't getting enough sleep at night, it will struggle to pay attention, will get easily distracted, will have trouble regulating other impulses, and will be less productive. And with ADHD, issues arising from poor sleep are further magnified. Stated plainly: If your brain hasn't gotten enough rest at night, it's not going to function well the next day. Poor and insufficient sleep negatively impacts all the core components of ADHD: attention and working memory, motivation, and impulse control. Moreover, in a kind of snowball effect, poor sleep negatively impacts many other brain functions, which can then also further exacerbate ADHD. For example, poor sleep negatively impacts mood, increases irritability and anxiety, and reduces the ability to access healthy coping mechanisms to deal with stress. These "emotional blocks" can in turn further impact a person's baseline ADHD challenges. So, someone who is operating on poor sleep not only has direct negative impacts from that on their core ADHD symptoms, but also has negative impacts from lack of sleep on other emotional and mental functions, which independently further worsen their ADHD. Poor sleep sets in motion an escalating cycle of negative impacts on your ADHD that, of course, will often further contribute to additional sleep issues.

One estimate is that somewhere between 25% and 50% of people with ADHD have poor sleep. This could be too few hours of sleep, but it also could be poor-quality/nonrestorative sleep. According to the National Sleep Foundation, the following numbers of hours of sleep are recommended:

- Children
  - Preschoolers (3 to 5 years): 10 to 13 hours
  - Kids (6 to 13 years): 9 to 11 hours
- Teenagers: 8 to 10 hours
- Adults: approximately 8 hours

Of course, these are average numbers, and some people need more or less than average. However, many people don't get as much sleep as they need, and that definitely contributes to poor focus during the day. To make matters worse, most of us are unaware how much this is impacting us. In general, people tend to overestimate their cognitive abilities when they are tired. They may think they are alert but perform poorly on tests of cognitive ability. The bottom line is that even if a person thinks they are OK while operating on less-than-adequate sleep, their ability to focus and manage tasks is probably still affected. So if you're going to see a doctor because you think you have ADHD, this is obviously very important.

Kids with sleep deprivation can still be hyperactive, so you can't rule out a sleep issue if your kid is energetic. And unfortunately, that could impact your own sleep!

Most people like to "sleep in" on some days (on weekends, for example), but this can contribute to a disturbed sleep/wake cycle, especially in people who are more sensitive to the effects of poor sleep. Sleeping in can make it difficult to fall asleep at an appropriate hour that night. It can also quickly snowball into increasingly disrupted sleep and additional sleep deprivation with each successive day.

The term "insomnia" means repeated difficulty falling asleep, waking up at night, or waking too early in the morning. Insomnia can be a symptom of conditions like depression, stress, and anxiety. Anxiety tends to make people have a hard time "turning their brain off at night" and initially falling asleep; it can similarly wake them up and prevent them from falling back asleep in the middle of the night.

However, many people with ADHD lose sleep for other reasons, including the following:

- ADHDers have trouble sticking to a schedule; this can contribute to sleeping in late and staying up late.
- Nighttime is when there are the fewest external distractions, and so it's also when it's easiest to stick to a task; some ADHDers stay up late to capitalize on this.

- Medications for ADHD can worsen insomnia (although paradoxically stimulants can improve sleep in people with ADHD, so long as they are taken early enough in the day).
- There is evidence from genetic studies that some of the genes involved in ADHD are also involved in sleep.

Medical Conditions

As with other psychiatric conditions, there are many medical conditions whose consequences can resemble ADHD.

Obstructive Sleep Apnea

Some people have poor-quality sleep for medical reasons. Possibly 15% to 30% of men and 10% to 15% of women have **obstructive sleep apnea**, which means that they do not breathe well while they are asleep. This is due to blockage or collapsing of the upper airways.

The risk of apnea increases when a person is overweight and also with age. East Asians, due to differences in facial structure, are at higher risk as well. Kids with big tonsils and adenoids are also at high risk for sleep apnea.

Snoring can be a sign of sleep apnea. However, not everyone who snores has sleep apnea (and some people not known to snore do have sleep apnea). Snoring reflects turbulent (that is, restricted) airflow through a person's nose and airways, resulting in less-than-optimal oxygenation of their brain while asleep. This can lead to many micro-awakenings throughout the night. That is, the person may not be aware they are waking up—they may not be fully awake or conscious at any time during the night—but their body repetitively jerks them out of deep sleep all night long, keeping them at lighter stages of sleep. Because of this, their sleep is nonrestorative. This can affect how rested they feel upon awakening in the morning and how well their brain functions the next day.

Nonrestorative sleep can lead to a variety of problems beyond ADHD. In addition to the mental and emotional consequences, it has other negative effects on the body. It has a negative impact on heart and lung function as well as on metabolism (it tends to increase stress hormones, leading to impaired glucose metabolism and difficulties with weight management).

Absence Seizures

Absence seizures are a type of **seizure disorder** (also known as **epilepsy**) occurring mostly in childhood that cause the person to have episodes during which they stare without consciousness. Most children with absence seizures eventually grow out of them, so this type of epilepsy is far more common in grade-school children and some adolescents than in adults. Absence seizures typically last around 10 seconds or less but can occur repetitively throughout the day. To an outside observer, it may appear that the child is merely daydreaming; because of this, absence seizures can make a child look like they are inattentive and have ADHD. In fact, children having absence seizures are extremely inattentive during their seizures and are completely unaware of anything going on around them—but this is quite different from ADHD.

So how does one tell the difference? Unlike a child with ADHD, who is simply staring out the window and daydreaming, children having absence seizures can't instantly be interrupted or "woken" in the middle of a seizure. Absence seizures also may disrupt a child at times or during events and activities when they would not be expected to be inattentive or daydream because of ADHD, such as while running or playing sports, in the middle of playing a videogame, or while doing other highly stimulating or pleasurable activities. Finally, absence seizures can (sometimes, though not always) be associated with unusual automatic body movements such as the head or limbs moving rhythmically, or the loss of bladder control (that is, the child may "wet their pants"). If you or your child's doctor have concerns about the possibility of absence seizures, the doctor should send your child for a brainwave test for seizures called an electroencephalogram (EEG).

Conditions that Cause Fatigue or Pain

Anemia is a condition where a person has low iron in their blood cells. This can be caused by a variety of different medical issues including poor dietary intake. Anemia often makes people feel like that don't have enough energy to do things, including concentrate. As ADHD is a lifelong condition and anemia usually develops later than childhood, these issues are not often confused, but anemia can contribute to symptoms of poor concentration. Similar to anemia, hypothyroidism is a medical condition that can cause people to feel fatigued and contribute to poor concentration. Again, it tends to develop later in life, and so while it is not often confused, it can certainly worsen ADHD symptoms. Chronic pain such as headaches (including migraines) can also contribute to poor functioning in people with ADHD. The pain represents another obstacle to overcome, and so can contribute to difficulty starting or continuing tasks. People with chronic pain also have increased problems with sleep, as well as increased anxiety and depression, all of which can worsen ADHD. Finally, medications taken for pain can make it hard to focus and concentrate.

As you consider whether you or your child have ADHD and whether it should be treated, be mindful of these conditions that can either mimic or worsen ADHD symptoms. Hopefully the professionals who are assisting you in this journey will be able to help you understand and address any of these issues so that your ability to function will be optimized. Any other caregivers involved should also be mindful that it may not be ADHD—or only ADHD—they are working with.

CHAPTER 6

Treatment with Medications

In this chapter, you will learn:

- How to decide whether and when to take a medication for ADHD
- General benefits and risks of medication treatment
- Types of ADHD medication and their specific benefits and side effects
- Supplements

What Makes It So Hard to Decide Whether to Take a Medication?

The decision over whether to take medication for ADHD may feel different from decisions you make about other medications for yourself or your family. If you have diabetes or high blood pressure, the medical guidelines are clear as to when a medication is needed—if you have such-and-such glucose levels or if your blood pressure reading is so high, there is near-universal professional agreement about starting a pill to treat the problem. Moreover, with these other types of medical conditions, the consequences of not treating the condition are very clear. Your doctor will tell you that if your glucose is not brought under better control, your kidneys, heart, blood vessels, and eyes will all suffer and ultimately fail. Similarly, if your blood pressure is not well controlled, your doctor will warn you that you have an increased risk of suffering a life-altering, if not life-ending, heart attack or stroke.

In contrast, when it comes to ADHD, as with other behavioral conditions, there are no numerical guidelines we or any other doctor can cite. No health care provider can say to you, "According to the American Medical Association, if your level of inattention is above this number, you should take this medication." So how are you supposed to know what to do? Should you start a medication when your child is getting C's, or should you wait for F's? If you're an adult, should you start a medication because you just got a bad performance review? Because you are somewhat more forgetful, inattentive, and stressed than your peers? Or do you wait until you've gotten fired from a job (or two) because of these problems? And what about non-medication strategies such as therapy or coaching—when should you consider them in addition to, or instead of, taking a medication? (We'll get to that more in Chapter 7.) The point here is that without a clear numerical test and guideline to go by, the provider's as well as the patient's and family's feelings and biases inevitably creep into the decision-making process of when and how to treat ADHD.

Compared to the medical examples given above, it may seem as though not treating ADHD has fewer negative consequences for the patient. No one will tell you that if you don't take a medication for your ADHD, you are going to die of a stroke, heart attack, or kidney failure. And yet this is somewhat of an illusion. As discussed in Chapter 1, there can be very severe consequences to not treating ADHD. It bears repeating that there are clearly identified, severe, negative consequences of not treating ADHD that include:

- Increased risk of motor vehicle accidents, concussions, and accidents in general
- Increased risk of depression, anxiety, and suicide
- Increased incidence of early pregnancy as well as sexually transmitted diseases due to impulsive behavior

- Relationship difficulties such as divorce and parenting problems
- Poor school achievement and therefore a less successful career trajectory and higher chance of poverty
- Increased risk for legal problems, bankruptcy, and criminal behavior
- Increased exposure to violence, both as a perpetrator and as a victim
- Increased risk of substance abuse
- Increased medical problems linked to poor impulse control and difficulty remembering to take medication
- Lower life expectancy due to all of the above

There is one more factor we wish to highlight that can make the decision of whether to take a medication ADHD more difficult. For everybody, when it comes to judging our own thoughts, feelings, and behavior, we are not objective. It can be very hard to evaluate either the source or the depth of our challenges. A chief reason for this is that the human brain, which is ultimately responsible for all our thoughts, feelings, and behaviors, is also a great illusionist. We are all extremely good at deceiving ourselves about the true inner sources of our problems.

With neuropsychiatric conditions, unlike other medical conditions, there is a tendency for people to believe that such issues can be corrected simply by "trying harder." There is also a tendency to "externalize" mental health problems—that is, to blame other people or circumstances for the problem. It is often very difficult for any of us to accept that the interpersonal challenges or other failures we may be experiencing have ourself as their main source. As for parents, making the decision to give a medication to their child may feel like a commentary on them, or like a personal failure. They might think, "My child wouldn't need medication if I were a better parent." The fear of social stigma also may play a role: Even if they themselves don't believe that their child's attentional difficulties are their fault, they may worry about what other people in their community might think (more on this below). Similarly, an adult may view needing medication for ADHD as proof they are a failure rather than as treatment for a legitimate medical issue. As for the consequences of not treating the condition, even if a health care provider brings up the list of potential bad outcomes, patients often think, "Well, none of that will never happen to me." A parent may find it hard to accept that their kid's school achievement might hinge on whether they give their child a medication. Additionally, many adults have difficulty accepting that they may need to take a medication to avoid things like getting into a car crash, falling victim to substance abuse, or struggling in their relationships.

For many, the struggle is entirely internal. Depending on how well you cope externally, the people around you may not know that you spent four times as long as you should have on something due to distractions, or that you procrastinated and did it all at the last minute—they just know you turned it in. So people in your life may discourage you from getting treatment or treating your child with medication. They may have the opinion that your issues are so minor that no medications are needed. All of these factors can make the decision to take medication less straightforward.

Another reason many people struggle with whether to begin medication for ADHD is the historical stigma and misconceptions associated with the diagnosis (as discussed in Chapter 2). The attitude that ADHD is caused by a moral failure ("bad kids with bad parents") still permeates many people's thoughts about the use of medication for ADHD, even if it is widely accepted that ADHD has a physiological basis. This is further complicated by the mistaken belief that the most common stimulants are highly addictive when prescribed for ADHD. Taking prescription Adderall for ADHD is falsely equated with using the highly addictive street drug "crystal meth," which, while also an amphetamine, has important chemical differences.

In short, choosing whether to take a medication for ADHD often diverges into the realm of emotional decision-making rather than being a logical assessment of pros and cons. With the following sections, we hope to take a little of the emotion out of this topic and discuss it instead as a more typical medical decision.

If you do decide to go forward with taking a medication, you should know you are not alone. Society is moving rapidly toward more medication prescriptions for ADHD, in stunningly brisk numbers. According to the U.S. Centers for Disease Control and Prevention (CDC), and also depending on the state, somewhere between 50% and 90% of kids with a diagnosis of ADHD are treated with ADHD medications at some point. Overall, about 70% of people diagnosed with ADHD try a medication for it. Between 2003 and 2015, ADHD prescriptions for adult women increased approximately 300% to 700%, depending on the age group (the highest change was in those aged 25 to 35). A recent study estimated that 6% (16 million) of adults in the United States had a prescription for stimulant medication (mostly for ADHD) in 2015 and 2016, an increase of 250% from 2006. Despite concerns from some quarters about "overdiagnosis" and "overtreatment," these numbers fit with expectations based on prevalence rates for the disorder in children and adults (see Chapter 1).

Addressing Parental Fears

Parents often bring to the appointment specific fears that may have been engendered by browsing the internet or talking to friends and that frequently are based on misconceptions. Among these is the fear that an ADHD medication will permanently change their child's personality or even permanently damage their child's brain. There is simply no evidence to support either of these beliefs. While it is possible that a child's mood will be affected negatively by either a stimulant or a nonstimulant, such changes are reversible. Mostly, mood should not change, or it may even improve. Generally, side effects stop when the medication is stopped. There is a very rare possibility that certain severe psychiatric conditions, like schizophrenia or bipolar disorder, could have a psychotic or manic episode *triggered* by taking a stimulant—but these underlying conditions are not *caused* by stimulant medications.

Another common fear is that the medications are addictive or hard to stop in some way. This is also not true. A medication for ADHD can be stopped at any time, typically without negative consequences (other than possibly a few days of fatigue from stimulant withdrawal, similar to people who stop coffee suddenly). That said, the ADHD symptoms that the medication held in check are very likely to resurface once a medication is stopped, albeit possibly with different consequences as the child may be at a different life stage at that point (see Chapter 10). If somebody with ADHD really doesn't want to take a medication forever, is there some way to avoid it? Yes! By simultaneously pursuing ADHD coaching or therapy to develop life skills to better manage their ADHD challenges, the ADHDer will be in a far better position to stop taking medications in the future (see Chapter 7).

What Can I, My Partner, or My Child Hope to Get out of Taking a Medication?

In general, medications help an ADHDer's brain focus more automatically and easily. People with ADHD typically feel calmer while taking ADHD medications. Patients often comment, "The noise in my head is quieter." What does this mean? A person with ADHD who takes ADHD medications typically finds that they are more able to sit still, pay attention, and focus on a single task or conversation. They may experience a decrease in intrusive thoughts. They may also notice a decrease in impulsive behaviors such as interrupting other people, in part because they can pay attention better and wait their turn without feeling they must interrupt to say something before losing track of their thoughts. They also describe being less prone to procrastination and distraction, being better organized and able to prioritize better, and therefore being more productive with their time. This often leads to secondary improvements in anxiety and mood, because they no longer feel so overwhelmed and have a greater sense of accomplishment at the end of the day.

Because medications for ADHD can decrease impulsivity, they can literally save lives. If you or an ADHDer you love is spending money they don't have, taking drugs or other risky substances, or getting into accidents, a medication can be lifesaving. This can be particularly important when it comes to curbing distractibility or emotional reactivity while driving.

In the best case, taking medication means for some people that for the first time in their lives they start to experience success and to build self-esteem around their accomplishments. Tasks that were so difficult before, and for which they previously experienced so much negative feedback, turn into things they can do. This can lead to entirely new concepts of what they are capable of achieving.

Medications always work best if the person for whom they are prescribed is on board with taking them. If you are a parent, you should emphasize to your child that you are not trying to change them as a person. You love them, and because you love them, you want to help them get onto a cycle of success.

The Decision to Take Medication

There are many reasons to try a medication for ADHD, but among the most important is when other strategies have failed to fix the problem. It is perfectly reasonable to try ADHD coaching or an ADHD therapist to learn to cope with the challenges of ADHD behaviorally—we *always* encourage that (see Chapter 7). However, sometimes coaching or therapy isn't enough, or doesn't work fast enough. Not infrequently, a person seeking an ADHD evaluation is doing so because they have reached a crisis: If you're facing bankruptcy or divorce because of your inattention and impulse-control problems, you need a solution that can help you quickly—and that's most likely to come from a prescription medication. And sometimes the challenges of ADHD are so difficult to manage that to even begin to use coaching or therapy, it is necessary to first start taking a medication.

Katie is a 33-year-old woman who comes to the doctor's office with a problem: Her husband has just left her and is planning to file for divorce. They have two school-aged children whom she will now have to care for single-handedly part of the time. She works in retail.

She is tearful and anxious during the doctor's visit, saying she doesn't know how she is going to handle it. She explains her husband's reasons for leaving center on her inability to manage both her work and home life. He has long taken on all aspects of their home: cleaning, cooking, helping the kids with schoolwork, keeping track of appointments, and so forth, and complains he has no choice because she is so "scatterbrained." She readily admits he is right: In grade school she was constantly in trouble for talking and disrupting class. She has always had difficulties with procrastination and organizing tasks—she barely managed to graduate high school and only completed a year of community college before leaving to join the workforce.

In the past she saw an ADHD coach who tried to train her in skills to cope with her challenges. He also recommended some apps and websites to help. She tried them, but they never really took hold or made a dent in her problems. She balked when he suggested she might want to consider seeing a psychiatrist and trying a stimulant medication.

The final straw for her husband came this past weekend. On Friday evening she went to an "afterwork social" where she committed a serious indiscretion with "some random guy" she met at the bar. Her husband found out about it from a text he happened to see sent by one of her coworkers, and he understandably "blew his stack." She wished she could blame alcohol but says she barely drank anything that evening. She also wishes she could say it was the first time, but that isn't true either. The truth is, she doesn't understand how or why it happened. She insists she loves her husband and her family; she was just out having a good time and somehow "lost control."

As ADHD represents a difference in some aspects of brain biology (Chapter 3), it makes sense to treat the difference with medication to alter the biology if one chooses. Fortunately, if you do decide to use a medication, there is a very good chance it will be helpful. The medications used to treat ADHD are among the most effective medications we have for any neuropsychiatric condition. While a medication will not "cure" the underlying issue, it will address the issue biologically in a way that helps the ADHDer manage their symptoms much more effectively.

As we mentioned in the beginning of this chapter, there are no clear medical guidelines for when to start a medication. This can sometimes contribute to disagreements between parents as to whether it's time to start one for their child. This situation can become very stressful. If at all possible, we highly recommend that both parents take some time to really understand the position of the other: why their partner objects to medication or really wants their child to be on medication. By discussing the situation fully, both parents will feel "heard" and have a better chance of compromise. Sometimes in the process one parent may realize that their decision is being made on emotional rather than rational grounds and change their mind.

Choosing a Medication

Whether it's stimulants, nonstimulants, supplements, or other types of medication that are not specifically for ADHD, you and your doctor need to carefully consider different factors. Sometimes, you (or your child) might prefer a particular form the drug comes in: liquid medications, chewables, patches, or capsules or tablets. You may have heard of a friend or family member who had particularly good (or awful) experiences with one medication or another. If there are people in the family who abuse drugs, you might want to avoid medications with abuse potential so those family members don't gain access to it through your prescription. The cost of medications is often a significant issue for many and should be discussed with your doctor. And, of course, you want to avoid unpleasant side effects.

Genetic Testing to Optimize Medication Choice

In Chapter 3, we emphasized that while science has a lot to offer regarding the genetics and biology of ADHD, there is even more about ADHD that scientists don't yet understand. It is not yet possible to "run a blood test" or "do a genetic screen" to diagnose ADHD (or just about any other psychiatric condition). The genetics contributing to the condition are too complex, and we don't have enough of the pieces of the puzzle in hand to draw any reasonable conclusions based on the results of genetic testing. But what about genetic testing to tell you which ADHD medication will work best for you?

Currently available clinical genetic testing can reveal a little about how likely you are to have a negative response to a medication; it does not tell you whether it will be effective for your symptoms. Your response to a given medication is related mostly to differences in your metabolism, but also to the particular protein makeup of your brain. As more is learned about the genetics underlying neuropsychiatric conditions, and as advancements are made in how these data are put together and analyzed, we believe genetic testing will become increasingly clinically useful with regard to ADHD. For now, though, we (as well as the U.S. Food and Drug Administration [FDA] and professional organizations like the American Psychiatric Association and the American Medical Association) don't recommend it routinely to patients. In its current form, genetic testing typically doesn't reveal much that we couldn't find out more cheaply and reliably by simply trying a few medications to see how you respond to them. Another problem is that the results of genetic tests can sometimes lead patients astray, prompting them to seek unnecessary changes to a medication that was working well for them or to avoid trying a medication that could work for them. That said, if a patient has the means and wishes to get genetic testing, the results should be considered in the initial medication decision-making process with the patient.

> Edna, age 43, has taken an antidepressant medication for years at a steady, low dose to help control anxiety and occasional panic attacks. She arrived at this medication after trying several others that didn't work as well for her. However, she is careful to only take it at a low dose, because whenever she has tried a higher dose in the past, even accidentally, it made her feel a bit "woozy" and sleepy for much of the day.
>
> Edna also has ADHD, for which she takes a stimulant medication at a high dose to treat her attentional challenges. She has never really experienced any side effects from it. She has noticed she is less sensitive to caffeine than most people—for example, she routinely drinks several espressos a day without getting "caffeine jitters," and she doesn't have problems falling asleep even if she drinks a caffeinated beverage in the evening.
>
> She decides to take a mail-in genetic test based on marketing claims that the test will tell her which psychiatric medications are best for her. She is confused when she gets the results, particularly because they say the antidepressant she is already taking is "not recommended" for her.
>
> Edna takes the test results to her psychiatrist to ask for an explanation, and he tells her that the genetic findings are mostly based on how she metabolizes medications. The genetic test says she shouldn't take her current antidepressant medication because the results showed she is a relatively poor metabolizer of that drug. Based on these results, the test predicts that Edna might experience more negative side effects from the drug. However, the therapeutic effects versus side effects from any medication are the result of an interplay between many variables. The fact is, the medication Edna is taking is working well for her—better

than others she tried in the past. Edna's doctor recommends she keep taking the medication at her current effective, low dose that hasn't caused her any adverse effects.

As for her stimulant response, the test predicts Edna has high activity of an enzyme responsible for eliminating norepinephrine, dopamine, and certain other neurotransmitters from her synapses. This fits well with her experience of needing high doses of stimulants to treat her ADHD, and is probably why she can take these drugs and consume caffeine at high doses and they never really bother her.

Overall, the genetic testing confirms what Edna and her doctor had already figured out over many years of trying different things—that she responds well to a very low dose of a particular antidepressant to control anxiety, while she needs rather high doses of stimulant medications to treat her ADHD. Incidentally, the test does also suggest that a dietary supplement, L-methylfolate, which corresponds to a naturally occurring chemical that Edna's body synthesizes poorly, may be helpful to combat depression, if that ever becomes an issue for her in the future.

What Kinds of ADHD Medication Are There?

New patients frequently ask which is the best medication for ADHD. It would be great if there were one medication that worked best for everybody, but unfortunately, there is no one "best medication" for everyone. On the plus side, at least there are a lot of options.

All FDA-approved ADHD medications can be divided into two types: stimulant medications and nonstimulant medications. Approximately 95% of people who take medications for ADHD take stimulant medications. These medications work immediately and do not need to be taken every day—both popular features. Although it may seem counterintuitive for drugs called "stimulant medications," most people with ADHD are not "stimulated" by these drugs; instead, a person with ADHD is more likely to feel calmer after taking a stimulant because of the positive effects these medications have on their ability to focus their minds and pay attention (they were originally named stimulants due to their effects on wakefulness). Methylphenidate (Ritalin), mixed amphetamine salts (Adderall), lisdexamfetamine (Vyvanse), and dexmethylphenidate (Focalin) are the stimulant medications most commonly associated with ADHD, though there are many other brand-name varieties and formulations, as discussed further below.

The nonstimulants approved for use in ADHD are guanfacine extended release (Intuniv), clonidine extended release (Kapvay or Onyda XR), atomoxetine (Strattera), and viloxazine (Qelbree). These work a little bit differently from the stimulants: Their effects build up in your body over time and do not wear off at the end of each day. This is a major difference from stimulants, and one that is helpful for some patients. Nonstimulants also do not carry certain stigmas associated with the stimulants—that is, of potentially addictive medications regulated by the government.

The differences between stimulants and nonstimulants can be distilled down to how the medications affect norepinephrine and dopamine, two neurotransmitters in the brain affected by ADHD (see Chapter 3). At the simplest level, you can consider the difference to be whether the medication acts at the "on" switch for attention in the brain or the "off" switch or whether it has an effect somewhere else in the control system for these neurotransmitters. All stimulant medications mostly act at the "on" switch: They cause brain cells to make and release more dopamine and norepinephrine at their communication terminals (synapses). As you can imagine, this leads to rapid effects on the brain circuits that rely on these two neurotransmitters. Accordingly, ADHDers who respond well to stimulant medications find that these drugs work rapidly to "turn on" their focus and organizing capacity.

In contrast, nonstimulants work by disabling the "off" switch, and so they lead to more gradual accumulation of these same two neurotransmitters over time. The result is that their effectiveness builds up over a few weeks to months, but once they are in effect, they work 24/7. These medications need to be taken every day for at least a few weeks (on average) before they begin to work. People are not supposed to take weekends off these medications; however, these drugs can generally be stopped easily—that is, without any serious withdrawal or discontinuation symptoms. Once stopped, the person eventually returns to the symptoms they had before they started the medication.

The bottom line is that the biggest difference between stimulants and nonstimulants is that stimulants work right away, for the day you take them, and wear off sometime during that day; in contrast, nonstimulants take longer to work, but once they start working they continue to work all day long. The effect of stimulants is analogous to that of caffeine: If you drink coffee, it wakes you up for a few hours and then the effect dissipates. The next day, in order to wake up, you must drink coffee again. In contrast, nonstimulants work more like antidepressants: You take them every day and begin to notice their effects weeks or even months out.

It's important to realize that regardless of whether you have the predominantly hyperactive, predominantly inattentive, or combined presentation of ADHD, the same medications will work for you. Your doctor will generally help you choose a medication not based on the "subtype" of your ADHD presentation, but based on other practical factors: how long the medicine lasts, the form it takes (pill, capsule, liquid, or patch), and whether your insurance covers it (often a big consideration). Also, some people take both a stimulant and a nonstimulant at the same time. They may take a stimulant for its immediate effectiveness, but also a nonstimulant because they find it helps them stay focused and productive even after the stimulant has worn off.

Side Effects of Stimulant Medications

The perfect medication would have tons of benefits and no side effects at all. Unfortunately, there are no perfect medications. Below are some possible side effects you should be aware of, starting with the stimulant medications. The most common side effects of stimulants can be summed up as "worse sleep, worse appetite, and worse mood."

Insomnia

Difficulty falling asleep is a frequent complaint that comes with taking a stimulant medication. But, just as some people can drink caffeine at any time of the day or night and still fall asleep, some people do not have this side effect. A practical solution, at least for medications that have short-acting effects, is to take the medication in the morning so that it does not interfere with bedtime. That said, somewhat paradoxically, many adults with ADHD who take these medications report that their sleep is improved (so long as they don't take them too late in the day). This is because the patient has been much more productive during the day, so they feel more fatigued at night, as well as more able to relax and enjoy a sense of accomplishment at the end of each day. They go to bed with less anxiety about tasks hanging over their heads and therefore sleep better at night.

Weight Loss

At the doses usually prescribed for ADHD, loss of weight is seldom a problem for adults, though it can be an issue in growing children. There are often simple, practical ways to manage this side effect, such as eating higher-calorie foods and increasing calories at breakfast (before the medication takes effect) and dinner (after it wears off). Lack of an appetite for lunch is not uncommon, which means it is important to have breakfast! It's thought that for children with ADHD, taking a stimulant medication can have a small effect on growth, but it's unclear how common this really is. Many experts believe that if weight is maintained at an appropriate rate, growth will not be affected.

Mood Changes and Irritability

Stimulants can also have undesirable effects on mood. The patient may feel sadder, angrier, more irritable, or more anxious. Sometimes these side effects are associated with the stimulant wearing off at the end of the day, especially in the context of poor caloric intake earlier in the day—that is, the patient suddenly gets tired and hungry at the same time, without the medication in their body to help with impulse control. More rarely, psychotic episodes (that is, hallucinations, delusions, paranoia, erratic or aggressive behavior) can be induced, most often by high doses, and typically in people who are already predisposed to these issues because of comorbid psychiatric issues such as bipolar disorder or schizophrenia. These are, of course, serious consequences that must be monitored, and are one reason why these drugs should be prescribed by a trained and experienced physician. For most such patients this would be a sign that they should not be on a stimulant medication at all. For a minority, it could be a matter of carefully adjusting the dose.

Increased Heart Rate and Blood Pressure

Other side effects can include higher blood pressure or pulse. If you have very high blood pressure to begin with, a stimulant may not be the right medication for you. The effects on blood pressure are typically small; on average, stimulants increase blood pressure by 2 to 4 mm Hg and heart rate by 3 to 6 beats per minute. These effects are generally short-term and reversible, but there is evidence from a large Swedish population-based study that long-term use of stimulants is associated with a higher risk of developing cardiovascular problems, including high blood pressure and arterial disease.

Because of the potential for these problems, patients taking these medications should have their vital signs checked regularly by their doctor. Patients can also monitor their vital signs themselves between doctor visits by purchasing a blood pressure cuff to use at home. The benefits versus risks of taking these medications should always be weighed carefully. For healthy children and young adults, this is seldom an issue that interferes with treatment. In our experience, it is extremely rare for a pediatric cardiologist to recommend against taking a stimulant medication for ADHD because of heart problems. On the other hand, older adults or patients with pre-existing heart problems or medical conditions should exert caution before taking stimulant medications for ADHD. Coordination of care with other health care specialists (such as, a cardiologist) is sometimes advisable to ensure that taking these medications will not exacerbate a potentially dangerous medical problem.

Addiction

There is a black box warning on the stimulant medications saying that they have the potential to cause addiction. They are classified as Schedule II narcotics—more addictive than benzodiazepines such as diazepam (Valium), lorazepam (Ativan), or alprazolam (Xanax). When injected, snorted, or otherwise consumed rapidly in high doses, these medications do have high addictive potential. However, studies have shown that when given as oral medications, taken as directed, and at doses typically prescribed for ADHD, there is a low potential for abuse. There is also evidence that when ADHD is treated effectively with stimulants, the risk of abusing other drugs such as cannabis or cocaine is lowered. In short, there is no basis to consider stimulants, given at therapeutic doses for ADHD, as "gateway" drugs that open the door to greater substance abuse issues. Furthermore, stimulant drugs are highly monitored at all stages in the United States: Production, sales, prescribing, and pharmacy distribution are all overseen and regulated by government agencies at both the state and federal levels with the goal to detect and curb any diversion or abuse.

Miscellaneous

The common side effects of taking any new medication—such as headaches and stomachaches—can of course also happen when first taking stimulants. Please discuss any side effects with your doctor: Often making a dose adjustment or changing the specific medication can help.

Types of Stimulants

A common misconception about stimulants is that they are all amphetamines. The stimulants approved by the FDA for use in ADHD can be divided chemically into two types. There are **methylphenidate**-based ones (for example, Ritalin and Focalin) and **amphetamine**-based ones (for example, Adderall and Dexedrine). Each type has lots of different variations. A simplified categorization is presented in Figure 6.1.

As you can see from glancing at the figure, there are both immediate-release and longer-acting forms of each of these

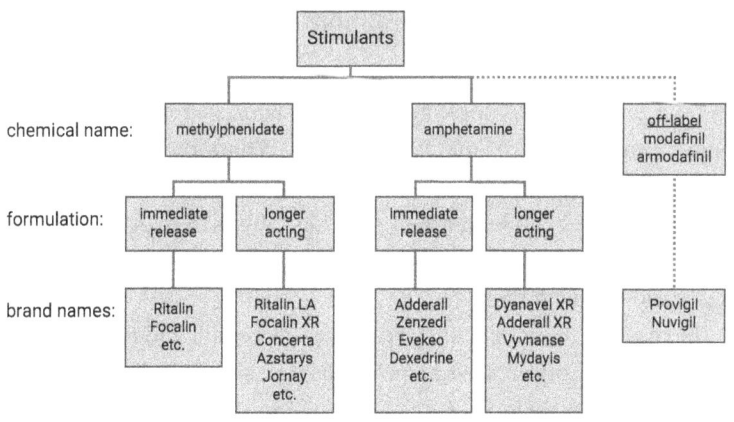

FIGURE 6.1 Relationships between stimulant medications for ADHD.

medications. As a rough guide, immediate-release stimulants work right away and last about 4 hours before their effects wear off. Most longer-acting formulations are designed to last about twice as long. However, you must take such numbers about duration with a heavy grain of salt, because different people have different metabolisms and often get quite different results. For example, we have patients who take a single immediate-release stimulant once in the morning and it lasts them the entire workday; these patients can't take a longer-acting formula at any time of the day or it will keep them up all night. We have other patients with fast metabolisms who take a longer-acting stimulant late in the morning or even early in the afternoon and still sleep just fine.

One reason why there are so many long-acting forms of these drugs is that different manufacturers have come up with different methods to slow-release the same active ingredient. Even though the active ingredient is identical, the different release mechanisms may work better or worse in individual patients. If one formulation works for you or your child but has undesirable side effects, another formulation of the same medication might be worth trying—it might work as well or better without those same side effects.

Methylphenidate-Based Stimulant Medications (Ritalin)

To take one example, look at Table 6.1, which shows the different long-acting versions of methylphenidate. What's the difference, you might ask, between Ritalin LA and Concerta? Well, Ritalin LA is a soluble capsule filled with little beads half of which release the medication right away, and half of which are coated so that they release the medication a few hours later.

In contrast, Concerta uses a different technology to achieve long-acting effects. Concerta has an insoluble capsule with a little hole in it, and inside the capsule, there is a little sponge. As your intestinal fluids seep through the hole, the sponge absorbs and expands, pushing

TABLE 6.1 Different Kinds of Short- to Medium-Acting Methylphenidate

Name	Generic Available?	Notes
Methylphenidate (Ritalin)	Yes	Lasts 3–4 hours
Dexmethylphenidate (Focalin)	Yes	Lasts 4 hours
Methylphenidate SR and Methylin ER	Yes	Lasts 4–6 hours
Metadate CD	Yes	Capsule lasts about 6 hours

methylphenidate out. The result is that about a third of the drug is released right away while the rest leaks out slowly over the next several hours. Both Concerta and Ritalin LA have the same active ingredient (methylphenidate) but because of this different release technology, they can have different effects in different people. Aptensio is a different brand of methylphenidate that lands in the middle: It releases 40% right away and 60% later on.

You can see from Table 6.2 that there are many long-acting methylphenidates. QuilliChew, Quillivant, and Cotempla are released more steadily over the day, using different technologies than Ritalin LA, Concerta, and Aptensio. QuilliChew is a chewable tablet, Quillivant is a liquid (with liquids, you can adjust your dose "to the drop"), and Cotempla is a dissolvable tablet.

So far, we've discussed tablets, chewable tablets, liquids, capsules, and a dissolving pill. There is also a methylphenidate patch called Daytrana that adheres discreetly to your hip. You put it on in the morning and take it off in the afternoon. It typically lasts about 9 hours or so.

There is another drug, Jornay, with a unique niche: It is a version of long-acting methylphenidate that is coated. When this drug is taken at bedtime, the coating dissolves overnight so that the active ingredient only starts to be released just before waking in the morning. The idea is that it works for ADHDers who have a particularly hard time getting going in the morning. It starts acting just before you wake up,

TABLE 6.2 Different Kinds of Long-Acting Methylphenidate

Name	How It Works	Generic Available?	Notes
Methylphenidate ER/Concerta	Releases 22% immediately, 78% over the day	Yes	Needs to be swallowed whole
Methylphenidate LA/Ritalin LA	Releases 50% early, 50% 4 hours later	Yes	Capsule that can be opened
Aptensio	Releases 40% early, 60% later	No	Capsule that can be opened
Daytrana	Releases over 9 hours	No	Patch
Cotempla	Steady release	No	Dissolves in the mouth
Quillivant/QuilliChew	Steady release, very long acting	No	Steady release, very long acting
Jornay	Taken at night, released first thing in the morning	No	Good for people who benefit from stimulants as soon as they wake up
Dexmethylphenidate XR/Focalin XR	Releases 50% immediately, 50% 4 hours later	Yes	This is a right-handed-rotation variation of methylphenidate.
Azstarys	Prodrug of Focalin	No	Body converts to active ingredient over the day.

so that you are ready to get up and get moving from the instant you open your eyes.

Dexmethylphenidate (Focalin) is a chemical "sibling" of methylphenidate (Ritalin). The difference between them is like the difference between your left hand and your right hand: the same structure, but mirror images. Methylphenidate means a mixture of both left- and right-handed molecules, whereas dexmethylphenidate (Focalin) means the right-handed molecules only. This matters for some individuals who respond differently to these two types of chemicals.

As with methylphenidate, there are both short- and long-acting forms of Focalin. Focalin XR is released 50% immediately and 50% around 4 hours later, similar in design to Ritalin LA. A newer medication, Azstarys, contains a "prodrug" for dexmethylphenidate—that is, as ingested, it is inactive. It needs to be metabolized to be converted into the active drug, which is dexmethylphenidate. This results in a more even release profile throughout the day that may help reduce negative side effects.

Amphetamine-Based Stimulant Medications (Adderall)

The amphetamine branch of stimulants includes mixed amphetamine salts (Adderall) and dextroamphetamine (Dexedrine), and both medications' long-acting forms. Adderall and Dexedrine have the same relationship to each other as methylphenidate (Ritalin) and dexmethylphenidate (Focalin); Adderall and most other amphetamine drugs are composed of both left- and right-handed molecules, whereas Dexedrine (dextroamphetamine) is composed exclusively of right-handed amphetamine. The left- and right-handed forms of amphetamine have slightly different effects on the release of dopamine and norepinephrine and can have subtly different effects in different people. The most commonly prescribed amphetamine is Adderall, which is composed of about 75% right-handed (dextro) amphetamines and 25% left-handed (levo) amphetamine. By way of contrast, Evekeo has about 50% of each, right and left (Table 6.3).

A long-acting form of Adderall is Adderall XR. As with Ritalin LA, it is designed so 50% is released immediately and the remaining 50% is released about 4 hours later.

TABLE 6.3 **Different Kinds of Short- to Medium-Acting Amphetamines**

Name	Generic Available?	Notes
Mixed amphetamine salts (Adderall)	Yes	Lasts 6 hours; 75% dextroamphetamine
Dexamphetamine (Dexedrine, Zenzedi)	Yes	Lasts 4–5 hours; 100% dextroamphetamine
Dextroamphetamine Spansules	Yes	Lasts about 6 hours; 100% dextroamphetamine
Evekeo	No	Lasts about 4–5 hours; 50% dextroamphetamine

Mydayis goes one step further: There are three layers to the beads inside the capsule, so it is even longer-acting than Adderall XR. As with the other soluble capsulated medications (such as Ritalin LA), even if you can't swallow capsules you can still use the medication by pulling the capsule apart and putting the beads on a spoonful of a soft food—but don't chew! (Chewing the beads releases all the medication at once so it is no longer a slow-acting medication.)

Similar to Azstarys, Vyvanse contains an inactive prodrug that must be converted by an enzyme in your body into the active stimulant, dextroamphetamine. This makes it last longer with a smoother "on and off" curve than Adderall or Adderall XR (Table 6.4).

Brand-Name Versus Generic Medication

Some medications, generally the newest, are only available as a "branded" version from the company that developed and patented it. If a drug has a generic form, this means the drug is older and that the patent has expired; many different companies can then manufacture the same medication, making it available at a cheaper price.

TABLE 6.4 Different Kinds of Long-Acting Amphetamines

Name	How It Works	Generic Available?	Notes
Adderall XR [=extended release mixed amphetamine salts]	Releases 50% early + 50% four hours later	Yes	Capsule can be opened; lasts about 8 hours
Vyvanse	Prodrug of major ingredient in Adderall (dextroamphetamine)	Yes	Body converts it to active drug over the day; capsule can be opened; lasts about 8 hours
MyDayIs	Very long-acting version of Adderall	No	Lasts about 12 hours
Xelstrym patch	Very long acting transdermally applied (non-oral) drug.	No	Lasts about 12 hours
Adzenys	Dissolves in mouth, releases gradually	No	Lasts 10-12 hours
Dyanavel	Chewable and liquid forms, gradual release	No	Lasts about 12 hours

Many people wonder whether to take the brand-name version of the medication or the generic. Newer brands are always priced much higher than generic medications. Generic options are supposed to be identical to the brand-name version, but the manufacturers are allowed about 10% leeway in terms of how close their formulation is to the original brand medication. For most people, this difference does not matter. However, the 10% discrepancy is enough to affect a small number of people adversely: They either don't experience as much of a benefit, or they experience greater side effects. Pharmacies can stock different generic manufacturers depending on what is available from wholesale suppliers. If you find you or your loved one are sensitive to one particular manufacturer, let your pharmacist know. However, you might need to find a different pharmacy that stocks the version that works best.

In general, newer branded stimulant medications are all variations on older medicines engineered to last longer, release more smoothly, and/or cause fewer side effects. If you're not sensitive to stimulant side effects, then you don't need to bother getting a medication that has fewer. For those who do find they need the newer medications, many suppliers have manufacturer's coupons available. Check online; the best ones are usually on the manufacturer's website.

Nonstimulants

There are four—or really two pairs—of FDA-approved nonstimulant medications for ADHD. The first pair are atomoxetine (Strattera) and viloxazine (Qelbree), which are mechanistically similar to each other. The second pair are clonidine extended release (Kapvay or Onyda XR) and guanfacine extended release (Intuniv), which are also mechanistically similar to each other (Figure 6.2).

In terms of common side effects, the nonstimulants are more likely to make you sleepy rather than keep you awake (though they may interfere with sleep as well), may cause nausea or gastrointestinal upset, and can have negative effects on mood. Clonidine and guanfacine can also lower blood pressure.

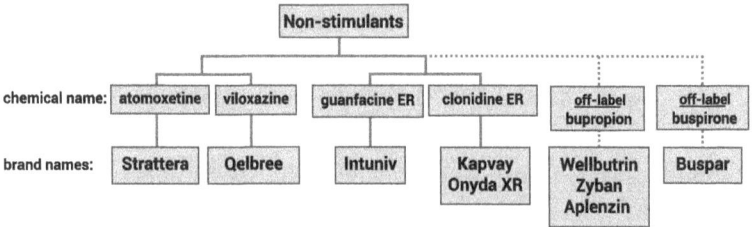

FIGURE 6.2 Nonstimulant medications for ADHD.

Like the stimulants, the first pair of nonstimulants (atomoxetine and viloxazine) increase dopamine and norepinephrine at synapses, but they do so in a different way from the stimulants. As stated earlier, these medications interfere with the "off" switch: That is, they interfere with a "sanitation system" that normally removes dopamine and norepinephrine once they have done their job at synapses. You could say that atomoxetine and viloxazine put this synapse sanitation system "on strike." Because cleanup is turned down, the neurotransmitters in the synapse stay there longer and build up. Compared to stimulant medications, these nonstimulants lead to more gradual and steady changes in the levels of dopamine and norepinephrine available. Accordingly, they lead to more gradual, but also more sustained (not just "as needed"), improvements in ADHD symptoms.

The other two nonstimulant medications, clonidine and guanfacine, work in a completely different way: They activate a subset of norepinephrine receivers (alpha-2A receptors) found abundantly in a part of your brain located behind your forehead (the prefrontal cortex). This part of your brain is important for executive decision-making: "paying attention to what's important while keeping a lid on distracting impulses." Activation of alpha-2A receptors by these medications strengthens connections in this part of your brain. This increases activity in executive decision-making circuits and leads to gradual improvement in some ADHD symptoms.

There are other differences between stimulants and nonstimulants that are worth mentioning. For one, your body is very good at removing stimulant medications. Remember, stimulants are out of your body (and brain) within hours of taking them, while nonstimulants (especially the first pair, atomoxetine and viloxazine) typically stick around longer. They build up in your system over a week or so, and if you stop taking them, they are eliminated over a similar amount of time. This contributes to the gradual onset (and offset) of their effects and correlates with patients' reports about their experience with these medications. Most ADHDers who respond well to nonstimulants find they work gradually and subtly (but nonetheless effectively) to improve focus and organizing capacity.

The forms of clonidine and guanfacine used to treat ADHD are engineered as coated pills or a specially formulated liquid (in the case of Onyda XR) to make them longer-acting, so they only need to be taken once or twice per day. The chemicals themselves are also available as short-acting forms, but to treat ADHD, they need to be present in the brain around the clock, so immediate-release forms are not very useful. Side effects are similar for both and have to do with their other major medical use as blood pressure medications. Too high a dose of either can lower blood pressure excessively, leading to a range of issues from lightheadedness at the mild end to fainting spells at the extreme end. In addition, both medications are slightly sedating, so some ADHDers prefer to take them before bed—that said, they also can sometimes interfere with sleep.

Off-Label Medications

Modafinil (Provigil) and armodafinil (Nuvigil) are two stimulant medications that are used "off-label" for ADHD. They are chemically distinct from other stimulants, and instead of being approved for treating ADHD, they have been approved to help people with certain medical conditions marked by abnormal sleep: narcolepsy, obstructive sleep apnea, and shift-work sleep issues. There have nonetheless been several studies showing that modafinil and armodafinil significantly reduce the symptoms of ADHD. Similar to the other stimulants, they are U.S. Drug Enforcement Agency (DEA)-controlled substances subject to special prescribing restrictions and controls because of concerns about their potential for addiction and abuse (although regulated at a slightly lower level). An important difference between these two stimulants and those approved for ADHD is that they have a longer duration of action.

Bupropion (Wellbutrin) is an antidepressant that has mechanistic overlap with the nonstimulants atomoxetine and viloxazine. It is a combined dopamine and norepinephrine-reuptake inhibitor. There is evidence that it can help alleviate the symptoms of ADHD, although it has not been FDA-approved for treating this condition. It is often seen as a choice for someone who is both depressed and has attentional issues, but it comes with certain downsides. For treating ADHD, it is often less effective than the FDA-approved medications, but because of its side-effect overlap (especially regarding heart rate and blood pressure) with ADHD medications, it may not always be safe to take both bupropion and a medication specifically for ADHD, especially another nonstimulant with a highly overlapping mechanism of action like atomoxetine or viloxazine. Unlike other antidepressants, but much like atomoxetine or viloxazine, it can cause increased feelings of edginess or anxiety and can interfere with sleep. Interestingly, because it also affects nicotine receptors, bupropion is FDA-approved as a smoking cessation aid. For ADHDers with a nicotine addiction who wish to kick the habit, this can be a side benefit.

Buspirone (Buspar) is less well known as an off-label treatment nonstimulant for ADHD, but there is some evidence it can be effective. It is FDA-approved for treating generalized anxiety and might be a good choice for people who have both anxiety and ADHD.

What about Caffeine?

New patients sometimes bring up their caffeine consumption in the context of "self-medication" for ADHD and/or concerns about potential overlap with stimulant medications. In research studies, caffeine has not been found to be a very effective treatment for ADHD. Why not? Caffeine (and its relative found in tea, theophylline) primarily affect a receptor in your brain for wakefulness. That is precisely why coffee, tea, and similar beverages are so effective for waking you up.

But unlike prescription stimulants, they have only secondary effects on the brain chemicals associated with ADHD. Accordingly, you have to consume a LOT of caffeine to produce similar therapeutic effects on attention as you get from taking a stimulant designed to treat ADHD—and by then you are dealing with unwanted side effects—i.e., the "caffeine jitters" that have the opposite effect on other domains of ADHD such as impulsivity and hyperactivity.

On the other hand, because caffeine acts like stimulants by increasing heart rate, blood pressure, and causing insomnia, care should certainly be taken when first starting a stimulant to moderate your caffeine consumption—at least until you know how the two chemicals work together in your system.

Dosing

"What's the right dose?" is an important clinical question. The dose that you and your doctor settle on is based on the balance of benefits (which should be high) versus side effects (which should be low). As stated previously, different people metabolize these medications at different rates. Fast metabolizers need higher doses. Slow metabolizers may experience benefits even with tiny doses. Unlike some other medications, the dosing of stimulant medication is not based on the patient's weight: There are many families where a fully-grown parent and their small child take the same dose of stimulant for ADHD.

The nonstimulants are somewhat different. Atomoxetine is dosed based on weight, and the dosage for viloxazine is mainly based on age (6- to 11-year-olds take a certain dose, 12- to 18-year-olds another, and adults yet another). As with the stimulants, it's harder to predict the effectiveness of guanfacine or clonidine based on a patient's weight.

Your doctor will likely recommend a "start low" approach to ADHD medications. Starting at too high a dose can lead to side effects that often complicate further treatment progress. Once started, the drugs can be increased in dose as needed, so it's important to be in close contact with your doctor when initiating these medications.

How Often Will I Need to See My Doctor?

Periodic visits for medication management are necessary to assess how the medication is working and where adjustments need to be made. Most medical doctors will meet with you every few weeks to every month or two in the beginning while first adjusting your dose. During this time, your doctor should be asking you about the resolution of your symptoms and adjusting your dosage accordingly. We recommend using a simple, quantifiable symptom rating scale at each follow-up visit to keep track of how the medicine is working for you. An example is the "Hyperactivity, Impulsivity, Inattention Symptom Rating Scale" (**HII-5**), which can be found in Appendix 2. The efficacy of the medication must be balanced against any side effects you may be experiencing. With stimulant medications, most people don't develop a lot of **tolerance**. This means that typically the dose that works best for you initially will remain pretty stable. It may require one final upward adjustment after your brain becomes fully habituated to it, but it should remain stable thereafter. Once you are on a stable dose of medication, your doctor will likely stretch out the time between visits as your need for any further medication adjustments will go down sharply.

Supplements

Some people wish to pursue a "natural" approach and use supplements rather than FDA-approved medications to treat their ADHD. Most supplements "don't hurt," but there is no supplement that helps ADHD nearly as much as a prescription medication. If a modest effect is acceptable to you, you can try them. The most common supplements include omega fatty acids, saffron, zinc, iron, and vitamin D.

There are other types of supplements called "nootropics." These are not vitamins, but a more diverse set of molecules meant to enhance cognitive function. Certain herbs such as ginseng and gingko are considered nootropics. Again, if you are after modest effects, they could be helpful. However, there are not, in our view, sufficient data regarding their efficacy or safety, especially in children.

Limitations of Medication-Based Treatments in Psychiatric Conditions

Even when medications work, they are not necessarily the whole answer for ADHD treatment. In fact, it has generally been found that what works best for treating psychiatric conditions is combining medications with non-medication approaches such as therapy or coaching.

As discussed in Chapters 4 and 5, ADHD is often comorbid with other psychiatric conditions, particularly mood and anxiety issues. This is relevant here because ADHD medications can sometimes exacerbate these other issues. Many ADHD medications can cause edginess and irritability and increase feelings and physical sensations of anxiety such as shakiness or heart palpitations. When these medications are taken by those who don't have ADHD or at too high a dose, these issues can cause big problems. But for those with ADHD, especially if their ADHD contributes to their anxiety or depression, properly treating ADHD with medication often improves these symptoms rather than exacerbating them.

Many people with ADHD are coping with external issues that contribute to their problems, including chaotic relationships, difficult social situations, and economic stress. It is critical to address these issues in order for a person to get better. As doctors who prescribe medications and other treatments for emotional and behavioral problems, we frequently remind adult patients that "Prozac won't fix your marriage," and kids that "Adderall won't do your homework for you." If issues in your personal life are contributing to your difficulties, a pill won't fix them; you need to work on them separately. This typically means working with a therapist or an ADHD coach.

It is plausible that therapy and coaching have more lasting benefits than taking a medication. Looked at this way, if you take medication without also learning new thinking strategies and behavioral skills to deal with your ADHD, then you have nothing to fall back on when the medication wears off at the end of the day or if you ever decide to stop taking it. That's like fertilizing a plant to make it grow but not staking it up so that it flops all over the ground.

On the flipside, as stated near the beginning of this chapter, there are patients who cannot make use of therapy or coaching until their worst symptoms are brought under some control with a medication. If you are too overwhelmed to use therapy because of your lack of focus, or because of the situation you have gotten yourself into due to your lack of focus (fired from work, flunked out of school, divorced from your partner, and so forth), then you may need to start with a medication. If you are so sensitive to criticism due to uncontrolled ADHD that you perceive every bit of constructive feedback offered by a therapist or coach as an attack and reject it out of hand, then you may need to start with a medication. The bottom line is, whether you can't use therapy or coaching because you are unable to focus long enough or because you are too emotionally sensitive, you may need to start by taking medication to address these issues first.

CHAPTER 7

Coaching and Therapy Tips

In this chapter, you will learn:

- How to use talk-based approaches for treating ADHD: coaching versus therapy
- Tips for managing ADHD behaviorally (with or without medication)

In Chapter 2, we discussed which types of professionals can diagnose ADHD. We talked about whether to go to a psychologist or a medical doctor, and also what kind of medical professional you could go to: nurse practitioner, primary care, psychiatrist, or neurologist. We also discussed different approaches to the diagnosis of ADHD. But wherever you go and however you are diagnosed, if you have ADHD, the next question is: What can you do about it?

Though there is no permanent "cure" for ADHD, there are many approaches to managing the symptoms, many of which are quite effective. For a long time, the mainstay of treatment has been taking medications, and these are very effective, as discussed in Chapter 6. Non-medication options for ADHD treatment have been increasing in recent years, particularly through the addition of technology-based approaches. Non-medication options should always be considered, as they can be effective and generally don't carry the burden of side effects that can come with taking a medication. That said, as with other behavioral conditions, it is usually true that the combination of medication plus non-medication treatment strategies is most effective for managing ADHD symptoms both in the short and long term.

Talk-Based Treatment Approaches: Coaching Versus Therapy

Once you've been diagnosed with ADHD, a range of mental health professionals can help treat it. When it comes to "talk-based" approaches, there is a basic division between "coaching" and "therapy." This division is partly historical and partly semantic. In a nutshell, "therapy" historically has referred to a range of talk-based approaches for treating many types of mental health problems. Therapy is most commonly practiced by psychologists and certain other types of licensed professionals, such as licensed clinical social workers (LCSW) or licensed marriage and family therapists (LMFT). Less commonly encountered therapy degrees include licensed professional clinical counselor (LPCC) and licensed educational psychologist (LEP). Some psychiatrists (medical doctors [MDs] or doctors of osteopathic medicine [DOs] with psychiatric specialty training, or alternatively PMHNPs) also do talk therapy as a part of their practice, typically in combination with prescribing medications.

Beyond the different types of professionals who do therapy, there are also many different types of therapy designed for different purposes and to treat different conditions. For example, there are specific therapies designed to treat panic attacks, phobias, post-traumatic stress disorder (PTSD), generalized anxiety, depression, and some kinds of personality disorders. One type of therapy that is broadly used and for which there is evidence for effectiveness in mood and anxiety disorders is **cognitive behavioral therapy** (CBT); it has recently also been adapted for use in treating ADHD (more on this below).

A confusing point for people seeking help is that individual therapists have individualized levels of training and competence with specific types of therapy, and this has little or nothing to do with their formal degree. Unfortunately, there is no way to tell by the degree behind somebody's name whether they are interested in or have experience or competence doing therapy for ADHD. So how do you find out? Well, you just have to ask them! It is of course also advisable to look at their website and read their online reviews.

Coaching, on the other hand, arose purely out of necessity around ADHD. One driving factor in the growth of ADHD coaching has been the shortage of therapists with an interest or expertise in treating ADHD. Coaches for ADHD may or may not have any professional degree or formal training. To take the dimmest view, anybody can advertise themselves as an ADHD coach and offer to take you as a client. That said, there are professional organizations that train and certify ADHD coaches, such as the ADHD Coach Training Center (iACTCenter.com) or the ADD Coach Academy (ADDCA.com). An ADHD coach is, by definition, someone who is focused on and interested in helping individuals and their families cope with the challenges created by ADHD. Many ADHD coaches bring a wealth of experience, expertise, and passion to what they do. Having someone like this "in your corner" can be an invaluable asset—whether you are an adult dealing with ADHD yourself, or a parent struggling to navigate how best to help your child with ADHD.

So, when it comes to ADHD coaching versus therapy—how do you know which to choose? First of all, it is important to note that these two approaches are not necessarily mutually exclusive and that you might want to have both. For example, if you are a parent of a child with ADHD, it might be ideal to have a therapist work with your child to help them learn better skills to manage their ADHD symptoms, while an ADHD coach works with you both to help you navigate practical issues created by ADHD in your home. For most people, this is not realistic either in terms of available time or financial resources. Among the clinical factors that may help you choose is if you have significant comorbid psychological issues, like depression or anxiety (see Chapter 5); they might also benefit from the help of a therapist.

That said, who you choose is most often a practical decision dictated by who is available and who is affordable. Coaches often charge less for their services than therapists, but their services are typically not covered by health insurance. On the other hand, your health insurance might theoretically cover the cost of seeing a therapist—if you can find one. The truth is that finding a therapist covered by insurance is often extremely difficult, verging on impossible, in many areas of the country. The economics of mental health care are such that many therapists simply don't want to work for the rates paid by insurance and so accept self-pay only. The result is that it is often very difficult and discouraging to try to find a therapist covered by insurance—let alone one who is also skilled in ADHD. Most people seeking this type of non-medication help with ADHD start by calling all the listed providers on their insurance company website, and then give up and turn to others—therapists and ADHD coaches—who are not covered by insurance and for whose services they have to pay out of pocket.

Types of Talk Therapy

As mentioned above, "therapy" is an umbrella term that covers a tremendous variety of psychological approaches for all types of mental health problems. Historically, the use of talk therapy to address mental health conditions goes back at least to Sigmund Freud, a neurologist who created **psychoanalysis** in the late 1800s and early 1900s. Psychoanalysis is a type of therapy in which the patient lies on a couch and free-associates out loud, while the doctor sits out of sight, taking notes and saying almost nothing. These days, psychoanalysis is not what most people mean when they talk about getting therapy for a mental health condition, and it's certainly not the type of therapy we mean when we talk about getting talk therapy for ADHD.

As mentioned above, a more modern approach to therapy that has been adapted for ADHD is cognitive behavioral therapy, or CBT. The "cognitive" in CBT refers to the way you think, while "behavioral" refers to the things you do. Indeed, the whole point of CBT is to learn skills to change the way you think and the things you do. In the case of CBT for ADHD, the point is to change the way you think about yourself and about situations where ADHD is affecting you negatively, and to change the things you do in response to those thoughts and situations. For example, if your ADHD has caused you to fail tests in the past, you may start to think of every test as a form of punishment that always has a bad outcome. This may make you anxious and discouraged before taking tests, and that in turn may cause you to do something counterproductive such as avoid preparing for the test. Of course, this cycle of thoughts and behavior inevitably leads you to have a bad experience on the test and to perform poorly, just as you expected. You conclude with the thought, "See, I'm a lousy test taker," and so the cycle continues.

A therapist performing CBT would start by helping the ADHDer identify their cycle of negative thoughts and actions. They would next work on changing how the ADHDer thinks about the test—after all, it's not really designed or intended as a punishment. They would work on helping the ADHDer make connections between how their negative thoughts and emotions about the test lead them to avoid preparing for it and encourage them to behave differently in the future. They would work on strategies to make studying easier, such as breaking study goals down into manageable steps and celebrating with some kind of reward each time a goal is met. The therapy might also include elements of CBT for anxiety and depression, since those are also factors in the above situation, helping the patient to find ways to lessen those negative emotions.

To look at another example, let's say you are an adult with ADHD who struggles with a lack of organization. Your partner is looking for an overdue bill and asks if you've seen it or moved it anywhere on the desk you share with her at home. You may have reached a point where, when your partner asks you such a question, you immediately perceive it as criticism. You think she is nagging you again about your chronic struggles with organization, even if she actually is just looking for that unpaid bill. So instead of responding appropriately, you feel hurt and resentful, and an hour later get into a heated argument with her about something unrelated. CBT might focus on helping you see the bigger picture—how your ADHD has led you to think in certain ways such as perceiving an innocent question as a personal attack. From there, it would focus on different ways you could have thought about your partner's question and different ways you could have responded instead. Perhaps you should have simply said, "No, I haven't seen it," and then asked if she would mind helping you organize the desk since it is not something you do well by yourself.

There is a variant of CBT called **dialectical behavioral therapy (DBT)** that can also be helpful in coping with situations like the one described above. DBT is intended to develop mindfulness, distress tolerance, emotional regulation, and interpersonal skills. It focuses a little more on identifying "triggers" (such as your partner asking you if you've moved anything on the desk) that tend to provoke a negative thought cycle and emotional state in you. The mindfulness component of DBT includes meditation, breathing, and other self-soothing and grounding exercises to help you become more aware of connections between your mental processes, emotional reactions, and bodily responses. The goal of this process is to decrease automatic or habitual negative thoughts, associated emotional reactions, and resulting interpersonal conflicts. With both CBT and DBT, the idea is to understand the mental wellsprings of your emotions and then reappraise how you respond behaviorally to them.

Children, especially those under 10 years of age, often do not do well with CBT, DBT, or other types of one-on-one talk therapy, because these approaches require a level of abstract thought and executive functioning they have not yet developed (see also Chapter 10). There are accordingly specific types of therapy designed to help children as well as their parents and families. In **parent–child interaction therapy**, a therapist observes a parent and child playing or working on a task together, discusses it with them, and then provides feedback about what took place and how the interaction might be improved. This is often coupled with **parent management training** from either a therapist or a coach, which is more directly focused on helping an adult learn better parenting skills. In much the same way that managers at a workplace should ideally receive training to learn how to get the best out of their employees, you as a parent might benefit from learning techniques that help you be the best parent you can be for your children, particularly if any of them are experiencing ADHD challenges. Finally, if your child has been struggling to get along in school with other children, **play therapy** is an approach to help them express and process their feelings, particularly if, for developmental reasons, they don't yet know how to do so verbally.

Some Useful Coaching and Therapy Tips

Depending on the background and expertise of your therapist or coach, they might work with you in a variety of ways, focusing on different aspects of ADHD, employing different strategies, and helping you develop different insights and skills to better cope with it. We cannot provide an exhaustive list of every therapeutic approach and skill a good coach or therapist might employ to help you with ADHD, but there are some therapeutic concepts and skills we've found helpful that are worth reviewing. These strategies will help you regardless of whether you also decide to take a medication for ADHD. As stated at the outset of this chapter and elsewhere in this book, what tends to work best is generally the combination of medication (as recommended by a doctor or nurse practitioner) and training in these types of skills with the help of a therapist or ADHD coach.

Set Goals

Setting goals is useful for everybody, but it is especially important for ADHDers. Goals must always be achievable, involve a reasonable plan for how they may be achieved, and come with a timeline and deadline. A goal without a practical plan, timeline, or deadline is just a dream or fantasy. When setting goals, it is critical to ensure that the goal is at an appropriate level of difficulty and immediacy for the individual. For an ADHDer who may have grown used to a lifetime of underachievement, it is important that goals not be too ambitious or long term, especially at first. Start by setting small, very achievable, short-term goals, and then slowly increase the difficulty and timescale of your goals as you get better at reaching them. A good strategy is to break large complicated tasks down into smaller achievable tasks that can be celebrated along the way (see also Chapter 8, on procrastination).

Goals also need to be adjusted for age. While adults may be able to work toward a long-term goal, for developmental reasons children generally need more immediate goals. The younger the child, the more straightforward the goal should be, and it should be paired with a very immediate reward once the goal is achieved (see also next subsection). Even a middle-school child, who may be old enough to appreciate the relationship between how they do in school now and thoughts of eventually going to college, may still not be equipped to respond consistently to the long-term goal of "academic or career success" alone; they need something more concrete and immediate to work toward.

Celebrate Each Success

In parallel with goal setting, it is important that each successful achievement, no matter how small, be celebrated and rewarded. This doesn't mean you have to throw a party every time your child manages to get his backpack ready or, for an adult, have an ice cream sundae every time you complete some mundane task—but it does mean recognizing that a goal has been met and congratulating the person who met it. Depending on the significance of the goal, the "celebration" can be as little as some words of positive recognition and encouragement or as much as a party with friends. But no matter what, it is crucial that it be recognized and celebrated.

> *Sam is a 37-year-old with ADHD and a busy life. Between kids, a job, his wife and her job, taking care of the house, and volunteering for the dads' club at his kids' school, he often feels he does not get any downtime. There is no end to his responsibilities; he's constantly being pulled in 1,000 different directions and continually falling behind. No matter what he does, something always falls through the cracks. He starts to get depressed. When he is depressed, he procrastinates more and falls even further behind.*
>
> *He does much better once he adopts the habit of giving himself a mental pat on the back whenever he finishes a piece of work. A simple "Good job, me!," at times coupled with another small personal reward, helps him see his tasks as more personally meaningful and fulfilling, rather than as just more work. While still very busy, he can motivate himself and feels more capable of doing what he needs to do.*

Celebrating success feeds into a virtuous cycle that we call the **cycle of success**: This is the cycle of behavior in which each success breeds more confidence and self-esteem, and more confidence and self-esteem breeds the desire to engage in further goal setting and achievement. Our brains are generally programmed to notice the negatives more than the positives in our lives—this is what psychologists term the "negativity bias" of our brains. To counter it, we have to make an extra effort to notice positives and celebrate successes. As a rough guide, it's best to recognize three good things you've done for every negative outcome you have. This is also true for giving feedback to loved ones with ADHD: They should hear about three positives from you for every corrective comment you make.

Visualization

Therapists and coaches often work with their clients to help them visualize the future as they wish it to be. This can be extremely important for helping someone with ADHD who has become discouraged from repeatedly not reaching their potential. Unlike goal setting, visualization does not require a plan, timeline, or deadline but is instead about having a long-term positive outlook about what is possible for you.

When using visualization, it is important to stay positive by working at imagining what achieving certain goals will look like. Visualize yourself finishing a project or help your kids to picture in their mind how they will feel when they get a report card with their desired grades. The more detailed and vivid you can make the visualization, the more effective it will be.

Positive visualization can be contrasted with visualization of a future in which the ADHDer doesn't change what they are doing right now. The point of this is to compare the consequences of acting versus not acting. Ask: "How will 'Future You' feel about 'Present You,' depending on what you choose to do now?" By bringing the consequences of the future into the present, the ADHDer is more likely to feel motivated to make changes and take action now.

Improve Time Management

Taking too long to do tasks and running late is a frequent problem for ADHDers. There are behavioral ways to address these issues, including the ample use of timers to develop a better sense of how long it takes to do things. To do anything faster, you need to know how long you generally take to do it and set goals to speed up (along with a plan for how you will do so). So, use a timer, but don't make the mistake of being too rigorous about the time taken to complete a task. Many people worry too much about "What if I'm not done when my timer is up?" Remind the ADHDer it is not a "fail" if they do not finish "on time." If the timer goes off before they finish, that is the cue for them to think it over: "Was I slower than I should have been, or did I set an unrealistic goal for how long the task would take?" If they are using the timer to develop a sense of time, then they shouldn't just turn the timer off if the task isn't done; they should hit "snooze" and keep going! Then they should record how long it actually takes them to complete the task—both as a way of developing a better sense of how long it takes them to do things and also to try to improve on this in the future.

Interval Training

"Interval training" means working in short, intense bursts and then taking a brief break. One technique for this is the Pomodoro method, which involves setting timers both for the length of time one is going to spend on a specific task and also for the length of time one will take a break from the task before getting back to it. These days there are a number of Pomodoro apps available; let your ADHDer choose the one that works best for them.

Many are designed to have work intervals of 25 minutes followed by a 5-minute break. After three such rounds, you get a longer break of 15 minutes. Of course, you can adapt this as needed; we recommend not being too strict about the exact length of each interval. The ideal interval of intense activity may be less—or more—depending on the age of the person and the task at hand. The idea is that it is better to read in a focused manner for 5 minutes at a time in four bursts than to spend 20 minutes reading in a unfocused manner. Though you are free to adapt the times involved, we do recommend not making the "breaks" longer than the "bursts." We also recommend doing something physical and/or easy during the break. For example, doing jumping jacks or running around the block is much better than playing a videogame or even pickup basketball with a friend, because it may be hard to stop and get back to work at the end of break time.

Identify Your Own Lies

Another important aspect of improving time management is learning to recognize your lies to yourself. Lateness generally arises from over-commitment, being distractible, hyperfocus, or miscalculating transition times. Often, the ADHDer is aware of these tendencies but repeatedly makes the mistake of telling themselves little lies to get around them. Here are some of the problematic self-deceptions many ADHDers tell themselves:

> *I'll get to that a bit later.*
> *I'll just check Instagram for a few minutes.*
> *I'll just straighten up my room for a while before I start my next task.*
> *I can do it myself. I don't need help.*
> *It'll be fine. I won't need my medication.*
> *I don't have to write that down; I'll remember it.*
> *I can do that later.*
> *I will be more productive after I . . .*
> *I'll just do this one little thing; then I'll leave (or switch tasks).*

A good therapist or coach can help the ADHDer learn to be more honest with themselves about these false statements and correct them.

Keep a To-Do List and Set Reminders

Avoid promising yourself you'll remember something later. When you find yourself saying, "I need to remember ___" and relying on your brain to do so, you should realize that even if that works, you are doing it the hard way. Remembering is hard, but writing tasks down or coming up with other ways to physically remind yourself is easy. For example, to remember to take your lunch to work, get in the habit of making it in advance and hanging your lunchbox on the doorknob that you use on your way out.

Practice Mindfulness

Mindfulness techniques intersect with the Buddhist principle of "be here now." They pull you into the present and help you focus on the moment. This is helpful for ADHDers because they tend to have a lot of regret over past mistakes, and these regrets can preoccupy them and prevent them from performing in the moment. At the same time, they also tend to worry over the future due to a lack of self-confidence borne out of their prior negative experiences. Mindfulness techniques include focusing on simple bodily functions that tie you to the present moment, such as breathing, maintaining your posture, and even smiling. Of course, you're not going to cure ADHD by standing up straight and smiling, but a slumped posture and a frown tells your brain that you are dejected and probably aren't focusing and working hard in the moment.

Remove Your "Self" from the Situation

A CBT technique called distanced self-talk can help people identify and work through difficult emotions by taking them less personally. The basic idea is to address yourself as "you" and try to describe your situation from an outside perspective. For example: "You think you are being rejected, but that might only be because you are overly sensitive to any form of criticism." Looking at a situation that is upsetting you from an outside perspective can help you be more rational and less emotional and reactive about it.

Practice Situation Selection Awareness

Situation selection awareness is a technique designed to help you understand how you sabotage yourself through situations you put yourself in, as well as those you avoid. For example, if you surround yourself with risk-takers, you are more likely to take risks yourself and get hurt. If you constantly overcommit due to impulsivity, that can lead to chronic lateness and being unable to deliver on promises.

> *Jahana, age 24, had always been friendly and energetic and seemed to have about a million friends growing up. She was so much fun that even though she was widely known as "flaky"—she often was very late to events or forgot to show up at all—her friends forgave her and kept inviting her out. Teachers in high school rolled their eyes when she walked in late, but she charmed them and never got into serious trouble.*
>
> *However, starting in college, this habit became less charming. Jahana was in four different organizations but often missed meetings for all of them. She started to lose the friends she made in those organizations as they bonded with the people who did show up. She really loved her boyfriend, but he broke up with her because she kept cancelling or no-showing for dates when she was distracted by other activities and commitments. She was often in a panic because she didn't do her schoolwork until the last minute, claiming she was "busy with her clubs." A panic attack was in fact what finally got her into the therapist's office.*
>
> *Jahana's therapist worked with her on identifying her values and making commitments only to the things that really mattered to her. He helped her see that although she liked joining clubs and "being involved," she actually only deeply cared about the goals of one of them. She reduced her involvement to that one club and actually spent energy on that. She committed to keeping her word, which made her feel better about herself. She finally started using a calendar and became much less "flaky."*

You may be someone who uses avoidance as a coping mechanism. Many people with ADHD have experienced a lot of criticism in the past for not achieving their goals and have internalized this and become very critical of themselves. Procrastinating on tasks or never starting them can be a maladaptive way of avoiding experiencing new internal or external criticism for poor performance. Understanding the sources of these behaviors, often with the help of a good therapist or coach, is a first step toward fighting against these tendencies.

Improve Communication Skills

ADHD generates a lot of challenges with interpersonal communication. People with ADHD have trouble paying attention when others are talking, and this naturally irritates other people. Also, since they themselves tend to wander off topic, other people have a hard time listening to them. Other people can get irritated with the tendency of those with ADHD, due to inattention or impulsiveness, to "say one thing but do another." People with ADHD have a lot to offer, but due to executive functioning issues, they have trouble with following through. To address these challenges, a therapist may work with members of the ADHDer's family along with the ADHDer themself. The therapist may ask family members to focus on positive interactions and outcomes and to strive to look at the ADHDer with a spirit of respect. Instead of emphasizing an ADHDer's failures, the therapist may encourage family members to take note of and emphasize what the ADHDer has done or is trying to accomplish. With the ADHDer, the therapist may work on recognizing when they are going off topic or speaking impulsively and learning to rein themselves in. The therapist may also encourage them to use specific words or phrases to avoid misunderstandings and clarify situations with their family. For example, the therapist may suggest that instead of saying, "You always criticize me," the ADHDer should use "I feel" sentences such as "When this happens, I feel ___."

Another strategy for improving communication is to "disappoint early." The impulsivity of ADHD makes it easy to overcommit and over-promise. As stated above, other people can get annoyed when the ADHDer says they will do something and then doesn't follow through. Instead, it's better to be very clear on what you are willing and able to do. Commit to the things you can realistically accomplish, but it's always better to admit you can't do something than to promise and then fail to follow through.

Couples Therapy

It is possible for a relationship to be very successful when one person has ADHD and the other doesn't, but ADHD can also be the issue that torpedoes a relationship. The non-ADHD partner may feel like they are forced to take on a "parent" role for the ADHD partner, while the ADHD partner may resent this and feel unappreciated. In this situation, couples therapy can be invaluable for helping each partner understand the other person's point of view and appreciate them.

Organization Therapy

Many (but not all) ADHDers tend to "leave a trail." They may often lose or misplace items or not put things away. This can get to the point where it becomes an enormous job for other family members to deal with.

If you are a parent or a significant other who likes their environment neater, you need to find a happy medium with your loved one who has ADHD. If you are the parent telling your child to clean up, they may or may not do it, but they will definitely be more likely to if they see the point in it. Remind your child that they don't like looking for things and that keeping things neat and organized makes it easier for them to find what they want. Turn it into a game: Instead of hanging up clothes, get some laundry baskets for the floor of your child's closet. Improve your child's basketball skills by seeing whether they can hit the laundry basket or the trash can from the "three-point" range. Make a fun "5-minute cleanup" time before bed, with music and laughter.

Adults may benefit from similar ideas, but sometimes a professional needs to be called in. There are professional organizers who not only help clean up a mess, but also set up systems to keep the mess from happening again.

Organization therapy can also focus on challenges specific to school. These might include things like organizing a backpack, breaking down big projects into smaller tasks, and managing due dates.

Rest and Relax

"All work and no play makes Jack a dull boy." We all need time to unwind with enjoyable activities. Relaxation recharges willpower and creativity, so make a real commitment to downtime. The ideal is to be able to relax and play without feeling guilty. A big problem for many people with ADHD is that they try to work for extended periods in a mode that's halfway "on" and halfway "off." This is usually not very productive and certainly not efficient. Whether you are an adult or a child with ADHD, a goal should be to work hard when you work, play when it's playtime, and not blend the two. Try to be either "on" or "off," not halfway in between. The "off" times are important and should be about recharging the mind and the body. Doing something active outdoors is often a good idea. And make sure to have fun!

Get Sufficient Exercise

Physical exercise is great for your brain. Regular exercise is good for the health of your heart, lungs, and blood vessels, and good health for these parts of the body is critical for the health and optimal functioning of your brain. Exercise also induces the production of natural signals in your brain that boost neuron growth, such as **brain-derived neurotrophic factor** (BDNF), and this increases working memory.

Regular exercise also reduces levels of stress hormones, thus reducing anxiety. Aim for at least 150 minutes of exercise per week. The type of exercise doesn't really matter, but it should be rigorous enough that it makes you sweat.

On a strictly practical level, for school-aged kids with ADHD, exercise in the form of organized sports can be a form of therapy in and of itself. A student playing a sport has to learn to follow the rules, respect other players, and be disciplined around training and time management. Student athletes often have to maintain a certain GPA to remain on the team, and they are penalized for missing practice. These requirements can be important sources of both positive and negative reinforcement, helping an ADHDer manage their symptoms.

Get Enough Sleep

Sleep problems go hand in hand with ADHD for many reasons. One reason is that sleep problems are tied to vicious cycles of behavior that arise in ADHD (for example, leaving tasks until the last minute, which often means staying up late the night before a deadline). Sleep problems may also be independently tied to the biology and genetics of ADHD (there is evidence that at least some of the genetics of ADHD overlaps with the genetics of poor sleep). As we discussed in Chapter 5, sleep deprivation is one of many conditions that can mimic ADHD, and it certainly is a condition that worsens it. Just remember: A brain that hasn't slept well is an unfocused, impulsive brain. Especially if you are struggling with ADHD, it is critical to work on optimizing your sleep and getting sufficient sleep on as regular a schedule as possible.

CHAPTER 8

Procrastination

A Major Problem for Most People with ADHD

In this chapter, you will learn:

- What procrastination is
- How to identify ambivalence
- Ways to understand the ADHDer's viewpoint
- Skills to manage procrastination

Procrastination

We are devoting a whole chapter to procrastination because it is such a common and problematic issue for people with ADHD. Procrastination is seen across the lifespan in ADHD, from childhood through adolescence and into adulthood. It is also one of the symptoms that people with ADHD find most frustrating. "Why do I procrastinate over and over?" It's worth thinking about: If you can figure out why you keep procrastinating, you may be better able to find a solution.

As a first step, let's consider why people with ADHD are prone to procrastination. To generalize, the brain of someone with ADHD has a harder time than average with things like prioritizing and focusing on one task for a long time. Compared to the non-ADHD brain, the ADHD brain tends to "see" the world "all at once." It may not take in all the details about any one thing, but it sees a little about a lot of things quickly. It actually does this by shifting attention rapidly between competing things—so quickly that at times it may feel as though it is doing it all simultaneously. Given that the ADHD brain is constantly shifting attention between many tasks and possibilities, it has more difficulty focusing on just one task to get started on.

A related reason why people with ADHD tend to procrastinate is that they are particularly easily distracted and "hooked" by tasks that have been designed to demand attention, such as modern electronics and recreational screens. When confronted about this challenge, many patients say, "I don't procrastinate because of the electronics; I'm on the electronics because I procrastinate." Either way, committing to putting extra screens away will make it easier to get started on the less compelling stuff. Of course, everyone plays and works on the same screens these days, so it isn't so simple to just put them all away. But there are many apps to help control one's electronic diet.

Another reason people with ADHD procrastinate is there is often just one little part of a task that keeps them from getting started. They want to put away the laundry but detest pairing socks, so they don't do it at all. They want to start their math but can't find their math book. The solution in this case is to identify the part of a task that keeps you from rolling forward and find a way to address that particular issue.

One of the most common and insidious reasons ADHDers procrastinate is that there are times when it actually works out pretty well for them. When they procrastinate and have to cram something in before a deadline, they become more efficient. Then they do in one day what someone else might take 2 weeks to do. It's just a short leap from there to get to "That's the only way I can work." Procrastination followed by working under intense deadline pressure becomes their "process." The problem is that sooner or later they get to a task that they can't get done at the last minute, and this becomes more and more likely as they move up in life. Sooner or later a person with this "method" gets advanced to a position where procrastination followed by racing to complete something at the last minute simply doesn't work and gets them into trouble with their subordinates, peers, or superiors.

It's important for ADHDers to identify whether the hidden positive reinforcement of "rushing" to meet a deadline is what is driving this behavior in them. If so, they then need to decide whether it's worth putting in the effort to get out of this habit in order to "take their game to the next level." That will mean learning how to get organized, how to work steadily according to a schedule, and how to consistently do a better job. The first step in this process is to uncover any hidden beliefs that they "must" work the way they always have.

Identifying Ambivalence

Someone who wants to do something but also *doesn't* want to do it is pulled in two directions. People in this state often wind up going nowhere. Having two competing "wants" is the definition of ambivalence. This is often a major reason why procrastination happens. If you sort of want to take out the trash but also don't want to get your hands dirty in the process, you are liable to put off your task. Getting rid of ambivalence by thinking of a solution to remove the undesirable part of the task (in this case, wearing gloves) helps with getting the task done.

Ambivalence often comes up when a person feels they should achieve something because of external pressure but doesn't care enough about it personally to actually work toward it. This is why it's so important, whenever a goal is set, to be clear about whose goal it is—and why it matters to that person. If it doesn't matter to the person working to complete the goal, then perhaps it's the wrong goal, or perhaps the person needs to find another way to think about it. In the above-mentioned example of taking out the trash, someone who feels resentful about having to do it may have a harder time coming to terms with it. If they feel their parents are making them do it, part of them won't want to simply because they are being forced. So what's a solution? If the person can reframe this chore as "Everybody in my family has chores. I am lucky to be part of a household where everyone contributes," that might make it more palatable. Another example is a common scenario for grade-school children: Their parents want them to get good grades, but the kids don't see the point. This leads to ambivalence and procrastination around studying. A solution here is to find a way for the kids to "buy in"—that is, by converting the goal so that it's not about getting a grade or even about academic performance, but instead about recognizing and appreciating the positive feeling they have when they do well.

For everybody, but especially for children with ADHD, it's important to be invested in the goal being worked toward. This is often a challenge and a source of interpersonal stress between kids with ADHD and their parents.

Understanding the ADHDer's Viewpoint

Sometimes parents will impose their viewpoint on their kids. For example, when a child is chronically late to school, to the kid it may just mean they have less school, which they don't like going to anyway. Being late for school is not as upsetting to that child as it may be for their parent who is late for work because they're spending time trying to get their kid to school every morning. Children, whether they have ADHD or not, tend to be focused on the immediate future, whereas an adult can think more abstractly and can consider long-term consequences. To give another example: Children know that the faster they finish their homework, no matter how poorly they do it, the sooner they can get to playing videogames with their friends. Meanwhile, their parents may be thinking about this quite differently: "If they don't learn to check their homework now while they're in fourth grade, they won't do it properly in high school either, they won't get into a good college, they won't get a good job, and then they won't have a good life!"

The point is that when considering how to motivate and work with people who have ADHD, whether a child or an adult, it's important to consider how they see the situation and what motivates them. Once you do that successfully, you can work to change that viewpoint or that behavior. In contrast, trying to impose an external goal or point of view on someone with ADHD will typically lead to more interpersonal conflict and frustration without improving outcomes for anybody.

> *Maurice, "Mo," had good grades in high school—his parents made sure of it. He had tutors, his parents were "on him" all the time about schoolwork, and he felt immense pressure to do well. His parents told him all the time that if he wanted a great job later in life, he needed to do well and go to a "good college." He did what they said; he felt he had no choice.*
>
> *Now at age 19, he wound up at the "good college," but about 2 months in, his grades tanked. He was doing a lot of fun activities—water polo, gaming clubs, and rooting for the team at weekend football and basketball games, not to mention hanging out at the dorms to talk to people and go to parties. The problem was that Mo could not really make himself study. He didn't have as many homework assignments as in high school, and he was given a lot less direction. He was simply given material in class and assigned reading and was then expected to somehow assimilate it before the midterm exam. If he thought about this at all, the concept seemed a bit magical to him—but who was he to question it? Midterms came, he pulled a few desperate all-nighters, but he simply could not make up for his procrastination and lack of preparation.*
>
> *When he talked about this cycle, he confessed to feeling sad, frustrated, and trapped. The truth was that to please his parents, he had chosen a major he didn't like and was attending a school he felt was academically too challenging for him. More pragmatically, he recognized he lacked some skills that many of his peers*

at college had. From grade school through high school, his time had been tightly structured for him by his parents. As a result, he had never learned how to make and stick to a schedule by himself, let alone how to prioritize important tasks among all the distractions that came with living among his peers on campus.

Skills to Manage Procrastination

Get Help with Your Personal Blocks

Is there one part of a task that is keeping you or your ADHDer from getting started and doing the whole task? Either outsource that one part of the task—for example, ask another family member to pair the socks while you sort the rest of the laundry. Hiring somebody just to help with a certain task may be an option. Finding a way to make a task easier or more palatable may be a good solution as well.

Start with the Smallest Bit

As the saying goes, "The journey of a thousand miles begins with a single step." Tasks seem overwhelming if you consider them in their entirety—this is daunting for anybody, let alone someone with ADHD (Figure 8.1). People who are successful at getting tasks done are good at starting with just the first step. For example, don't think, "I have to get all my taxes finished today"; rather, tell yourself, "I can just put my name, address, and social security number on the forms." If even that's too much, try, "I can load the forms on my computer" or "I can print out the forms" or even "I can touch my computer keyboard." For a child with ADHD, the equivalent might be "I can put my name on the top of my homework" instead of "I have to get the whole thing done in one sitting."

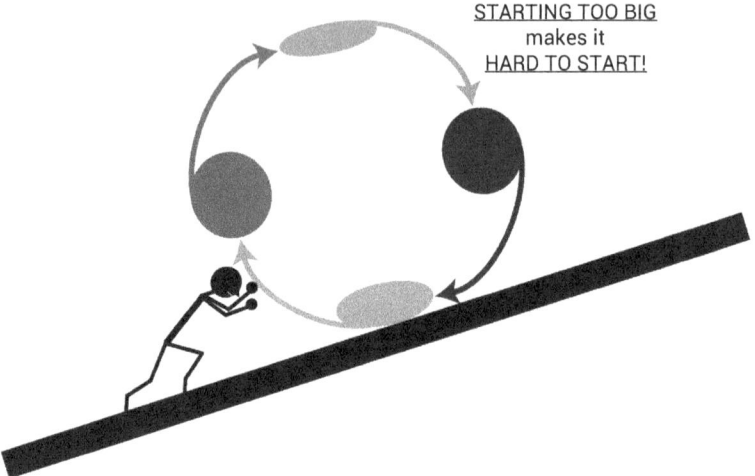

FIGURE 8.1 Starting with a task that is either too complex or too big often leads to failure to get started. (This graphic is taken from *ADHD & The Focused Mind*.)

Break Large, Complex Tasks Down into Smaller, Achievable Chunks

One of the principal causes of procrastination is being overwhelmed by large, complex tasks that you don't even know how best to begin. In these cases, it pays to plan: Break complex tasks down into the smallest achievable steps or chunks. Then make a to-do list with each of those smaller chunks as an individual goal. Celebrate each time you achieve an intermediate goal and take a break before moving on to the next one. This leads to a sense of accomplishment and builds self-esteem, which makes it easier to take on subsequent goals (Figure 8.2).

Schedule Dreaded Tasks Early

It's always tempting to simply avoid tasks you don't want to do. This is true for everybody, but ADHDers are often the worst offenders.

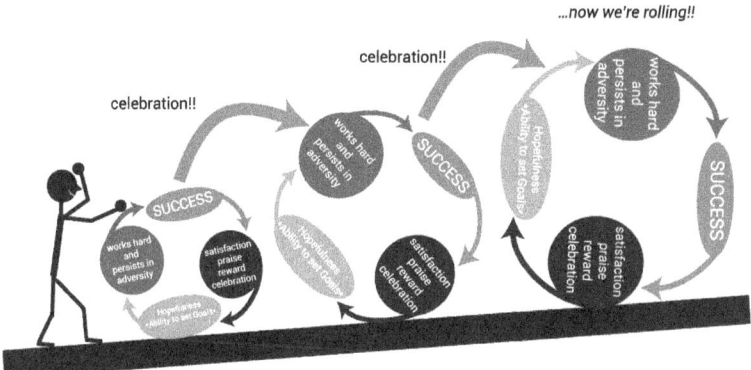

FIGURE 8.2 One antidote to procrastination is to break big, complex tasks into smaller, easier-to-accomplish steps, then celebrate each time you complete a step. This builds a repetitive cycle of success and improves self-esteem as part of a virtuous cycle. (This graphic is taken from *ADHD & The Focused Mind*.)

One approach is to very purposefully adopt the opposite habit: Do dreaded tasks early in the day rather than putting them off to later (which often means never). They don't have to be the *first* things done, because some people find that they become "paralyzed" by the thought of having to do those things and can't make themselves start. If that's your challenge, a more effective strategy may be specifically scheduling a dreaded task as the *second* item to get done, after completing an enjoyable task (or at least a less-dreaded task) first. This way you can ride the momentum you've built up, making it easier to tackle the dreaded task.

Setting a regular time to devote to these tasks every day is another approach. Earlier in the day is typically most successful as you'll have a higher reserve of energy to do the task. But no matter when you schedule it, remember that it's important to take time to give yourself or your loved one credit and celebrate when they complete one of those dreaded tasks. Doing so reinforces the habit of getting the hard things done, as well as helping to counteract any guilt they may carry around about tasks they previously had a habit of putting off.

If you are able to recognize that some activities are "sticky" (meaning it's hard to stop doing them) and some are "slippery" (meaning it's easy to get distracted and slip off them), you can schedule your time to have the highest chance of success. Try to get the slippery activities done when you think you will be most motivated to do so, which is often when you are best rested or after an exercise session. Try to schedule the sticky activities for when you have lower energy reserves.

Recognize and End "Procrastivity"

Procrastivity is an invented colloquialism that means doing something that's useful but shouldn't be done now, as a way of putting off what you should really be doing (but don't want to do). For example, an adult with ADHD might start organizing their bedroom closet when they are supposed to be working on their taxes that are due tomorrow. Of course, organizing the bedroom closet is not a "wrong" or "bad" thing to do—but why start on it now when their taxes are due tomorrow? For schoolchildren the equivalent might be working on an extra-credit assignment instead of the homework due the next day.

Why does this happen? For many ADHDers, the task they have gotten diverted to is mentally easier to tackle than the one they are putting off. Frequently, the diversionary task is one that's manual and that doesn't require a lot of mental energy, such as vacuuming, doing the laundry, or cleaning. Recognizing that this is what the ADHDer is doing is the first step in learning not to do it.

Impose Negative Consequences for Inaction

In general, positive rewards are more effective motivators than negative reinforcement, but there can be a place for the latter. The flipside of positive visualization and goal setting is to consider the negative consequences of inaction. Adult ADHDers may find it helpful to impose negative consequences on themselves for not completing tasks as scheduled. This is generally not needed for children with ADHD, as this type of reinforcement is usually already "baked in" to their schooling—often too much so. That said, although middle schoolers and high schoolers get frequent grades, younger children (who generally don't get grades) may need to get feedback from teachers more frequently if they have ADHD.

For adults, imposing consequences can be more effective than waiting for natural ones to happen, particularly as the latter might be far more severe (such as getting fired). As with goal setting, it's generally best to come up with consequences that are more immediate, frequent, and manageable. Make the consequence about something relevant to you right now—for example, you're "not allowed" to get yourself a little reward until you finish the page you are working on. Making a consequence external—that is, getting other people involved—can help a great deal. For example, to prevent lateness, tell a coworker you will buy them lunch whenever you're late for a meeting—or make it into a contest: Whoever is later buys the other one lunch. Adults with ADHD may want to request more frequent feedback about their work from their supervisor—this can help keep them honest with themselves about any problems or bad habits they engage in and avoid a worse outcome later.

> *Jason (age 45) frequently "forgot" to take the trash out (a chore he didn't like to do anyway). His family was irritated with him every week. To combat this, Jason let his family know that he would do extra cleaning chores such as mopping the floor whenever he forgot. This artificial consequence helped him get the job done, because the natural consequence of not taking the trash out was just "someone else does it," and that was far less motivating.*

In general, we believe that the best solution to procrastination, besides considering the above, is to simply practice *starting*. Never say, "I'm going to do it in 10 minutes," because that is practicing procrastination—it's literally practicing *not* starting. Remember, you get better at everything you practice. So practice starting instead—even if it's just by doing the tiniest possible bit of the task. If your task is to write something, maybe the way to start is just to open the document—or if you've done that already, maybe it's putting your name or a title at the top of the page. If the task you're stuck on is paying the bills, walk over to the pile of paper bills and just sort it, putting the oldest bills on top. The important thing is to make a start, even if it's just a little one.

Manage Electronic Distractions

Get serious about using app blockers to create blackout times for your electronic devices. If you say you spend too much time online but resist using a blocker (or are always deactivating it), you need to ask yourself why. Realistically, not all of us can avoid using screens as most of us need them to get our work done. Even so, they are the source of the most common, and compelling, distractions.

Managing screens is a skill that can be learned. If you are the parent of a younger child, it's essential to start early. When your child wants to have time on screens, ask them how long they think they should be on. That will probably be longer than they should be on, so try to negotiate for an agreeable time. Then ask the child: "How will you know when the time is up?" Show them how to set a timer. When the timer goes off, see if they can stop playing without being asked. If not, work on that. Through this process, you are showing your child that screens should not be without time limits. At the same time, the child is practicing the ability to end their time on the device themself. Make sure the child knows they have power over the device rather than vice versa. In our clinical practice, we ask, "Who is the boss of the phone? Are you bossing your phone around, or is the phone bossing you around?"

As teens get older, screen time can be even harder to manage. Not only are screens a gateway to the land of amusing videos, they also become part of their social fabric. But there are still approaches to limiting screen use that can be effective. One solution is installing software that limits how long your teen spends on their devices. Another could be a physical "handing in" of the phones at a certain hour in the evening. Another strategy, which also makes use of the "imposing negative consequences" tactic above, is to impose limits on a teen's screen time only if their grades start to dip.

No matter how you manage your child's phone, two elements are important to remember. First, no one will listen to you telling them to put their phone down if you yourself are always on your own device. Second, for safety reasons, impress upon every family member the importance of not using the device while driving.

As an adult, it's up to you to manage your own devices. Don't rely on willpower if you know that is a battle you or your child usually lose. Turn off notifications, close unneeded windows, and delete distracting apps. Then find electronic management software that helps you manage your screen time.

CHAPTER 9

Help in School and Self-Directed Treatments

In this chapter, you will learn:

- What supports are available for schoolchildren with ADHD (504 plans, IEPs, and other accommodations)
- What self-help strategies are available for ADHDers (blogs, vlogs, books, support groups, and other resources)
- What apps, websites, and other technology-based resources can help ADHDers

Help in School: 504 Plans, Individualized Education Programs, and Other Accommodations

Schools cannot "fix" a child's ADHD, but given that school is a particularly difficult place for children with ADHD, schools can make reasonable accommodations to help these children, at least temporarily. Not all students with ADHD will require extra help, but those who do can really benefit from it. Students and their families can ask for accommodations such as extra time to complete tests, allowing the student to take tests in a low-distraction environment such as on their own in an office, or allowing some leeway to turn in homework or projects after the deadline. By making accommodations, schools can significantly reduce stress on kids who are having difficulty performing well due to their ADHD. Of course, it can be difficult to walk the line between easing stress while also maintaining clear academic standards. It is important for parents to understand the options for accommodation that are available at their child's school, as school is such an important part of kids' lives, and school performance contributes not only to future prospects but also to self-esteem.

In public elementary, middle, and high schools, many children with ADHD qualify for a "504 plan." The name of this plan is an abbreviation for "Section 504," referring to the relevant section of the Americans with Disabilities Act (originally the Rehabilitation Act of 1973). Section 504 prohibits discrimination based on disability in programs or activities that receive federal financial assistance from the U.S. Department of Education (that is, all public schools). With a 504 plan, a student with ADHD may be eligible to get extra time (usually 50% more than the standard allotted time) on tests and to take tests in a low-distraction environment. Examples of other accommodations provided through a 504 plan might include leeway to turn in (at least some) homework late or being seated in a low-distraction area of the classroom. The child may be assigned to take a special class to help with organization. The goal of a 504 plan is to provide the child with a learning environment conducive to their needs. Having accommodations approved by the school administration takes decision-making out of the hands of individual teachers. Thus, if your child happens to get a teacher who doesn't "believe" in ADHD, having accommodations approved by the administration overrides the teacher's viewpoint.

Compared to a 504 plan, fewer children qualify for an individualized education program (IEP), which involves specialized instructions for the student. This is covered by the Individuals with Disabilities Education Act (IDEA). An IEP is a detailed plan that provides a child with individualized and specialized services at their school. For a child to get an IEP, they must qualify under one of the 13 conditions specified in the IDEA (such as blindness, deafness, autism, or specific learning disabilities such as dyslexia). ADHD can count, but in and of itself does not mean the child will get an IEP.

Both 504 plans and IEPs are free of charge to students and their families.

Children who attend private school may still qualify for help through their school district, but the private school is not held responsible under the rules of Section 504 or the IDEA laws. Special help for ADHD within a private school is administered at that school administration's discretion.

For additional information, see Appendix 1, Further Resources, at the end of this book.

Are Accommodations a Good Idea?

Accommodations provide you or your loved one with a modified school or workplace environment to address the disabilities created by ADHD. Without accommodations, some children with ADHD may work and work and work and still not succeed because the deck is stacked so high against them. If a child has repeated bad outcomes despite trying hard to succeed, it can hurt their self-esteem, make it difficult for them to maintain good intentions, and even lead them to just give up. Accommodations help even the playing field so that the student with ADHD can compete more effectively with their peers. That helps them feel better about school, build hope in themselves, stay engaged, and keep putting in effort.

On the other hand, some accommodation plans can be so accommodating that they backfire and fail to help the child. Children who are given too much leeway to turn in homework late won't be motivated to develop skills they need to turn in homework on time. When developing a plan, it's best to consider your "goalposts." Where do you want your child to be? If they are only turning in 50% of their homework on time now, perhaps the goal of the accommodation should be to help your child improve to 70% in 3 months and 90% in 6 months.

And what about after a child leaves high school to go to college? Many colleges offer accommodations for students with appropriately diagnosed and documented ADHD. Parents must discuss this with their child before the child leaves home. It's important for parents to portray their child's ADHD in an affirmative light and focus on what the child can do well, while helping them find appropriate mental health providers that will be accessible to them while they are at college. For instance, during orientation, schools will typically give out a phone number "in case you need mental health support." We recommend that parents make sure their child enters it in their phone for ease of access.

> *Mikaela, a 14-year-old ADHDer, had just started high school when her grades plummeted. She had previously been able to keep up with her work, but in seventh and eighth grades there hadn't been as much work assigned, so when she procrastinated or just plain didn't turn in her homework, there wasn't much in the way of consequences; she often still got A's. However, in high school, there was much more work as well as much larger class sizes, and Mikaela couldn't keep up. Her grades dropped and she was afraid and embarrassed to ask for help. She became stressed and figured she would never be able to make it in college, so she quit trying and then everything got worse.*
>
> *Mikaela and her parents met with school officials. The school gave Mikaela accommodations that included 150% time on tests and the ability to take tests in a separate classroom away from others. As a result she was no longer distracted by other people getting up, coughing, and turning in their tests while she was still working on hers, and was able to use the extra time to double-check her work and made fewer "silly errors." One of her classes became "resource room" where she got extra help with organization and time management. She was also allowed to turn in some assignments late without them being marked down.*

> Because her parents didn't want that to lead to a bad habit, it was noted as part of Mikaela's 504 plan that the number of late assignments allowed would decrease each trimester.
>
> As a result of these accommodations, Mikaela regained hope for her future. She started putting in more effort—and mostly succeeded. She was able to drop the resource room after a year and developed some new time management skills that helped her go on to be a successful college student.

Accommodations at Work

Recently, it has become more common for adults with ADHD to request work accommodations based on the American with Disabilities Act. It's unclear how this trend will evolve. There are certainly reasons why an adult with ADHD might benefit from some reasonable accommodations at work to help them maintain productivity, but we can also see some challenges and downsides for employers. We recommend patients discuss this issue with their human resources manager at work as well as with their doctor.

Self-Help: Blogs, Vlogs, Books, Support Groups, and Other Resources

ADHDers and their families often take heart from knowing they are not alone. They may feel alone as they grow up, not understanding why they are struggling. Finding out that there is a physiological explanation for what's been troubling them is validating. More and more sources of information about ADHD become available all the time. Resources such as blogs, podcasts, webinars, vlogs, and support groups offer support and can benefit you and the ADHDer in your life.

Electronic Aids (Apps, Websites, and Other Tools)

There are some electronic management aids that can help manage ADHD symptoms. A common symptom of ADHD is forgetfulness, which might include, for example, forgetting tasks that need to be done or forgetting appointments. Memory and attention employ similar circuitry in the brain, so ADHDers often have some difficulties with tasks that require remembering things. The idea behind these electronic aids is that they keep ADHDers from having to remember things. By setting a timer or a reminder, the person doesn't have to rely on their memory to retain all of the information related to a task or responsibility. For example, smart speakers can be used to create reminders or alarms with simple voice commands. Calendaring apps can also be an essential tool for setting notifications about upcoming events.

Electronic aids can also be used to manage blocks of working time. For example, Pomodoro apps use a time management method in which there are blocks of work time each followed by a short break (see also Chapter 7). Using a timer can help keep these blocks from spilling over into one another. There are many customizable timer apps that can be adapted for this method.

One of the most common types of electronic aids to help manage ADHD are apps that block distracting websites. ADHDers, especially those with high degrees of impulsivity, can deploy these apps to block access to websites they tend to use to distract themselves. See Appendix 1, Further Resources, for examples.

Technology-Based Treatments for ADHD

There have been attempts to harness the same technology that gives us all more distractions in the form of videogames to help manage ADHD symptoms. A videogame system called EndeavorRx has been approved by the U.S. Food and Drug Administration (FDA) for use with a prescription to improve ADHD in children. A similar game, EndeavorOTC, has been approved for use without a prescription in adults. Skylar's Run, a competing system made by a different manufacturer, uses a similar approach. The basic idea is to create a videogame that trains the player to pay attention and avoid distractions. The game adjusts depending on how well the player performs over time. This strategy works, but to be effective the game does need to be played regularly: The makers of the Endeavor games recommend playing at least 25 minutes per day, 5 days per week, for at least 4 consecutive weeks to see improvements in attention. While that may sound attractive to someone who likes playing videogames already, keep in mind that nothing makes a child *not* want to play a game as much as telling them they have to. It may be challenging to adhere to this prescription (or enforce it on a child) in practice.

A different type of technology, called **trigeminal nerve stimulation** (TNS), uses superficial stimulation of one of the main nerves in the face to improve ADHD symptoms. It's self-administered at home, nightly, while a person sleeps. It has been approved by the FDA as a treatment for ADHD in children but not adults. This device appears to be particularly helpful for improving some of the executive function issues in ADHD. Both TNS and the videogame approach work about as well as nonstimulant medications for some aspects of ADHD. And much like a nonstimulant medication, they must be used regularly to remain effective.

Another technology, called **transcranial magnetic stimulation** (TMS), treats mental disorders by using a fluctuating electromagnetic field to increase or suppress activity in selected brain regions and circuits. In the United States, TMS has so far been approved by the FDA for treating depression, anxiety associated with depression, **obsessive–compulsive disorder** (OCD), migraine headaches, and for smoking cessation. Recent incarnations of TMS use either an electroencephalogram (EEG) or functional brain imaging to target treatment to the specific brain regions showing abnormal activity in an individual patient. This is the first example of an FDA-approved use of brain imaging to optimize treatment for a psychiatric condition. TMS has pro-cognitive effects—that is, patients getting TMS often notice that after treatments they can think more clearly—and it has been investigated (though not yet approved by the FDA) as a treatment for ADHD. It is exciting to speculate that an individually tailored approach using functional brain imaging to target TMS could one day prove useful in ADHD.

CHAPTER 10

ADHD Across the Lifespan

In this chapter, you will learn:

- How ADHD is different in children versus adults, including biological factors (such as brain growth and a person's sex) and psychosocial factors (such as the influence of school, work, and the family)
- How therapeutic approaches differ for children versus adults
- How differences across the lifespan affect diagnosis in children versus adults

How ADHD Is Different in Children Versus Adults

ADHD is now recognized as a lifelong disorder. Because it often affects adults and children in the same families, and because many parents of kids with ADHD have concerns about their own ADHD, we have discussed ADHD in both children and adults in every chapter of this book. For the most part this works, because ADHD—including its symptoms, challenges, diagnosis, and treatment—is far more similar than different in children and adults. But that doesn't mean ADHD or the concerns it raises are completely static over a lifetime. This chapter specifically addresses how ADHD is different in children compared to adults.

Biological Factors, Part 1: The Developing Brain

First, let's talk biology. A baby's head circumference averages 13.75 inches (35 cm), while an adult's head circumference is about 50% greater, averaging 22 inches (56 cm). Most of that difference in head size has to do with the brain inside; a baby's brain is far smaller than an adult's. But is a human baby's brain simply a smaller version of an adult human's brain? The simple answer is "no."

Brain growth reflects a number of normal developmental processes. One of the main processes driving brain growth, especially **in utero** and during early infancy, is the birth of new brain cells through cell division. By the time a human baby is born, their brain has 100 billion neurons, meaning that on average during pregnancy, 250,000 neurons are created per minute. This is even more remarkable when you consider that is only the average over 9 months: that is, there are periods during pregnancy when brain cells are being created much faster than that. The creation of new brain cells through cell division was a factor driving the growth of your own brain and head until you were about 1.5 years old, when the total number of neurons inside your skull reached its maximum. Brain growth through cell division contributes less and less after the first year of life as other developmental processes take over. These processes include the growth and increased complexity of existing brain cells. During infancy, our brain also grows and becomes more complex by adding more **synapses** (which, as you may recall from Chapter 3, are the specialized communication zones between your neurons). Existing synapses also become larger and more structurally complex. This developmental process is concentrated in the first 2 years of life, peaking only a few months after brain growth through cell division. In fact, the overall synaptic density in your brain reached its maximum when you were about 2 years old and has been declining ever since. This is because the addition of new synapses is counterbalanced by an opposing developmental process called synaptic "pruning," which is the removal of synapses that are no longer needed. The process of synaptic pruning is most important developmentally throughout childhood and early adolescence—that is, from the ages of 2 to 16. A final major developmental process contributing to brain growth in later childhood and adolescence is the laying down of communication pathways between brain regions and their insulation through **myelination**. This insulation process allows brain regions to communicate with each other more quickly, facilitating more efficient brain circuits and networks (see also Chapter 3).

It is very important to stress that the synopsis provided in the preceding paragraph is a vast oversimplification. For one thing, while the basic sequence and timeframes we have provided for these developmental processes are essentially correct, they do not take place everywhere in the brain simultaneously or at the same rate. To look at an extreme example, the birth of new neurons through cell division continues far into adulthood in some brain areas (for example, the hippocampus, part of the limbic system and default mode network) many years after this process has effectively ceased in other areas of the brain. Moreover, for the brain to operate correctly as a whole throughout the various stages of your life, these developmental processes must be tightly coordinated within and between brain areas. Human brain development is a truly remarkable, complex, and highly orchestrated and choreographed affair.

The result of all the choreography between these developmental processes is what we observe as increasingly complex thought and behavior as we grow up. The human brain at birth is only a basic brain—it's been put together just well enough to ensure survival, and it only accomplishes even that much with a lot of help and protection from parents and family members. The newborn brain can use its senses to look around, listen, and feel; it can coordinate body movements involved in crying, eating, swallowing, breathing, regulating heart rate, peeing, and pooping—and that's about it. As it grows and adds biological complexity through the developmental processes outlined above (adding more neurons, making more complex connections between them, eliminating connections that aren't useful, and forging more efficient long-distance communication between brain regions), it gains correspondingly more complex abilities. Toddlers can understand language, talk, walk, reach for what they want, and start to develop an understanding of cause and effect. As children mature further, they make gains in physical and athletic abilities, become more creative, and eventually learn to read, do math, and engage in increasingly abstract and logical thought processes.

Among the core cognitive abilities affected by ADHD, executive functioning (the ability to plan, pay attention, remember, and juggle multiple tasks) is the last to emerge because it is the most complicated. It requires complex brain networks that only develop as the brain becomes more mature. The ability to use executive functioning skills typically begins in late childhood but continues to develop through adolescence and beyond, even into a person's 20s. This contrasts with some other types of human behavior that emerge earlier in development, such as basic emotional processing and responding to drives that yield immediate gratification. In biological terms, this creates a gap during normal development when brain regions involved with emotions and gratification are fully assembled and raring to go, while brain regions involved with executive functioning are still being assembled.

To summarize, infants, children, and teens are not simply "little adults," and this reflects the normal process of brain development. As we age, our brains change. The brains of kids and teens, because they are still developing, are organized differently than those of fully mature adults.

As mentioned in Chapter 3, there is a model that attempts to explain ADHD as a disorder of development in which the brain areas involved in executive functioning, such as the right prefrontal cortex, take a bit longer than normal to mature relative to other brain areas, such as those involved in generating emotions, drives, and impulses. This model has been supported by at least one research study in which children with and without ADHD had repeated scans of their brain anatomy over many years. This model could explain why at least some children with ADHD do seem eventually to "grow out of it." Against this, recent epidemiological research suggests that most kids with ADHD do not "grow out of it" and that features of ADHD persist into adulthood in approximately two-thirds of cases. This suggests that ADHD cannot be explained, in most of the children who have it, as a delay in brain development that "catches up" later. For most people ADHD is a lifelong disorder. Nevertheless, the fact that a child's brain is put together differently than an adolescent's brain, and that an adolescent's brain is put together differently than a fully mature adult's brain, is relevant to ADHD, because it contributes to how ADHD looks different and has different consequences at different life stages.

Biological Factors, Part 2: Sex and Gender

There is another aspect of biology that cannot be avoided when discussing ADHD: sex and gender. "Sex" in this case refers to male versus female biological differences, whereas "gender" refers to male versus female self-assigned roles and societal expectations. Both are important and cannot be avoided because historically, ADHD was more commonly diagnosed in school-aged boys than girls, and there is a lingering misconception both in the lay public and even among some professionals that ADHD is a diagnosis mostly afflicting grade-school boys. The most recent U.S. government survey statistics continue to show that ADHD is more commonly diagnosed in male versus female individuals. Yet a growing body of clinical and research evidence suggests that the true rate of ADHD across sexes/genders is much closer than historically thought.

As described in Chapter 2, ADHD was originally identified by pediatric specialists and educators of grade-school children because it interfered with schooling. What did it interfere with exactly? At the youngest ages, children are not expected to pay attention for long periods of time, follow complex directions, or work independently.

They are expected, within certain parameters, to listen to their teacher, follow simple directions, sit quietly or nap for at least short stretches of time, get along with other children, and not engage in risky activities that can cause harm to themselves or others. It was interference with these activities that brought young children to the concern of teachers and school administrators and ultimately to pediatric specialists.

The chief concerns of teachers and parents bringing the youngest school-age children in for evaluation have traditionally been issues with hyperactivity and impulsivity—behavioral challenges that lead to disciplinary problems in class or to risky behaviors on the playground. To this day, these types of concerns are more likely to be identified in little boys than little girls. The extent to which this reflects underlying biological differences in brain development in boys and girls, versus cultural biases affecting how little boys and girls are perceived and taught to behave, is open to debate, and we won't try to settle it here. What we will focus on instead is that as boys and girls proceed through grade school and as expectations rise among their teachers and parents that they should be able to pay attention longer, follow more complex instructions, and accomplish a greater amount of work independently, so too does ADHD diagnosis start to equalize between boys and girls. Just as it's slowly been recognized over the past few decades that ADHD is a lifelong disorder that can change in presentation at different life stages, so too has recognition grown that ADHD may present differently for many other reasons, including the expectations society places upon the individuals—of any gender—who have it.

The closing of the gap in ADHD between genders is nowhere more evident than in adults, and this likely has a cultural basis. In industrialized societies, women are often not only the family's "bread bakers" but also the "breadwinners." Many women hold down two full-time jobs: one at home and the other in the workforce. Here are a few relevant statistics for the United States:

Women, including working women, are roughly twice as likely as men to handle all the household responsibilities.

Women are three times more likely than married fathers to keep children's schedules and get them to their activities.

Sixty-three percent of women have missed work to care for sick children or because school is closed, versus 29% of men.

More women than men (59% vs. 32%) say they oversee ensuring all the household needs are handled.

Women also handle a lot of the "invisible tasks" in the family: remembering who likes to eat what, sending birthday greetings to relatives, tracking school-related tasks, and so forth. Women are also more likely to oversee other types of family scheduling, such as vacation planning, pet care appointments, buying presents, preparing thank-you gifts for teachers, meeting with household workers, or just watering the plants. Even by itself this represents a lot of work for one person to handle; combine it with also holding down a job outside the home and you have a "perfect storm" for someone with ADHD. Given this situation stemming from how our society is organized, it should surprise no one that adult women are increasingly seeking help from the medical community to cope with feeling overwhelmed, anxious, and depressed because of challenges with task management and executive functioning. This brings us to the next section.

Psychosocial Factors, Part 1: School and Work

As alluded to in the previous sections, it is deceptive to discuss the biology of the human brain as though it is divorced from psychology or society. When it comes to the brain, biology, psychology, and social functioning are all just different ways of looking at the same thing. That is, psychology and social functioning are reflections of the biology of our brains as they function individually and collectively. Moreover, just as our brain biology affects our psychology and social functioning, the reverse is also true: Our individual psychology and our social functioning are constantly impacting each other and our underlying brain biology as well.

When it comes to ADHD, what this means is that the challenges of the disorder change as a person progresses through preschool, grade school, high school, college, and then into work life and other aspects of adulthood—not only because of changes in brain biology but also because of changes in psychological and social factors at these ages.

Preschool

Parents, teachers, and the rest of society don't really expect a whole lot from preschool children when it comes to paying attention in class or keeping track of their personal items. At this age, what tends to draw ADHDers to the attention of teachers and parents are physical impulse control issues. Developmentally, little kids tend to be at their most active during this stage of life, and so the consequences of ADHD at this age are often directly related to the hyperactive and impulsive aspects of the disorder. These kids are often known as the "troublemakers" in class or in the family (and at this age, it's hard to get a medical diagnosis to explain their behavior). They have a hard time sitting still and may talk too much and distract other children.

The playground is another place these kids often get into trouble. Lack of structure on the playground can bring out their worst. They may have trouble waiting their turn or waiting in line. They may "butt in" to other children's games. They may get angry and slam a ball at another child in frustration. They may climb to the top of the monkey bars and jump off, or jump from other heights that tend to make playground monitors anxious and upset, even if it doesn't lead to physical injury. They can also be more prone to other types of impulsive behavior such as lying or stealing.

Already at this early age, the social consequences of ADHD begin to be felt. Teachers are more often angry at the child who disrupts class. Other children in class will take cues from the adult; some of them get annoyed and side with the teacher against the child with ADHD because the child is "being bad." In general, kids with ADHD at this age wind up hearing many, many "no!" statements. Though exact estimates vary, most psychologists agree that, at least when it comes to developing a positive sense of self, there is an optimal ratio of hearing positive statements to corrective statements at a young age. As mentioned in Chapter 1, if that is three positive statements for every one negative statement, children with ADHD often wind up hearing the reverse or worse: 30 negative statements for every positive. If you grow up hearing other people tell you that you are always doing the "wrong thing," you eventually come to believe it. Your motivation to do the "right thing" becomes low, because doing "right" is the opposite of your self-identity.

Elementary School

As children progress from preschool to grade school, expectations rise for them to be able to play together in larger groups. This includes playing games on teams according to increasingly complex and inflexible rules (think of organized games and leagues of baseball, soccer, or football in contrast to going on slides or climbing structures on the playground). Meanwhile, classes become more structured and demanding as well. As children progress through grade school, they are expected to pay closer attention, follow increasingly complex directions from their teacher, and work independently or in small groups for longer stretches of time and with more ambitious goals.

Coincident with these changes in expectations, parents and teachers of grade-school kids tend to raise concerns about children who have difficulty paying attention in class as well as challenges with hyperactivity, controlling impulses, and other discipline issues that may have been evident earlier. The negative statements continue to pile up.

Middle School

As children go on to middle school, their parents' level of control over them goes down. Many parents give middle schoolers access to their own phone, and with that comes the challenges of managing electronic distractions. That's a big challenge even for adults let alone middle schoolers. At a time when kids are insecure about their own self-image and may feel more pressure from schoolwork and extracurricular activities, their phone provides a convenient escape. As difficult a challenge as this may be in general, it is multiplied for the middle schooler with ADHD.

Middle school also demands an exponentially increased degree of organization compared to elementary school. In most middle schools, children have different teachers assigning different work in different classes, and they must organize and prioritize their homework themselves. They have to keep track of different school supplies and papers as they move to different classes. They must find a way to get the right homework to the right teachers on time. Tasks like these are challenging for many middle schoolers, but can be excruciatingly so for those with ADHD. This is further exacerbated by the generally larger class sizes in middle school compared to elementary school. Middle-school teachers cannot assist individual kids with their organization as much as they might have in elementary school.

The 2 to 3 years of middle school can be a time of intense personal growth. By their eighth-grade graduation, middle-school children have changed a great deal—both physically and mentally. Both boys and girls experience intense physical growth and changes. They are given more personal responsibilities at both school and at home. Many girls are getting used to having periods and the emotional ups and downs that can come with a menstrual cycle, which can in turn affect their ability to get their schoolwork done. Concerns about emerging sexuality are often far more important than math grades to kids at this age. The physical awkwardness that most middle schoolers experience can sideline children with ADHD even more, as they already tend to have poorer self-esteem compared to their peers.

The middle schoolers' changing bodies and the increasing attention paid to their bodies often comes with increasing demands on their time to take care of their bodies. This, combined with the general tendency to procrastinate plus increasing academic expectations (including long-term projects, which are easier to procrastinate on), means middle schoolers with ADHD may lose more sleep than their peers and experience decreased focus as a result. An ADHDer with poor impulse control (often combined with poor self-esteem) may fight with peers more—and by middle school, kids are getting big and strong enough to really injure someone. Middle school is also a time when many kids are first exposed to the temptations of trying drugs and alcohol, and due to their impulsivity ADHDers are more likely to try them. In short, the trouble ADHDers tend to get into in middle school is often much more severe than in elementary school.

High School

As children with ADHD move into the high school years (ages 14 and up), executive function issues, such as difficulties with prioritizing work, staying organized, and avoiding procrastination, tend to come to the fore as the concerns most often raised by teachers and parents. The pace of learning is faster than in middle school, so the consequences of falling behind are more devastating. It is at this age that kids with ADHD often develop their most severe challenges when it comes to coping with the academic workload.

If a younger child had 20 minutes of homework that took them three times that long to complete due to procrastination and distractibility, they, their parents, and their teacher might not have even noticed, or may have been able to cope and adapt without seeking a diagnosis or other professional help. In middle school, an hour of homework turning into 2 hours is still doable and might still be rationalized away. However, in high school, when 2 or more hours of homework each night divided between many subjects takes 4 to 6 hours to complete, it seriously disrupts time for everything else, including sleep. Not only does the high schooler simply have a greater amount of work to do, but completing that work efficiently requires organization, planning, and prioritization. The child who could cope with 20 minutes of homework becoming an hour due to their inattention becomes the teen who can't get 2 hours of homework done even if they allot more than 6 hours to it every day. Aside from the direct consequences this has on grades and academic achievement, it also leads to downstream effects that feed a vicious cycle of unproductivity and unhappiness. More time on homework means less time for extracurricular clubs, sports, other forms of exercise, social activities, and sleep. Not least of all, it leads to a resentful attitude toward schoolwork, which the child grows to view as the root of all their problems. This attitude may not end with high school—it can last a lifetime.

Some parents at this stage intervene by monitoring their high schooler's work very aggressively. That can work in the short term, but often leads to other problems later. Psychologically, it often contributes to simmering resentments between the child and the parents, and that may come out down the road. And sooner or later the child must inevitably move out from under their parents' watchful eyes and function on their own. This is when they discover they don't know how.

It is important to stress that as children get older, even as academic expectations change and increase, the challenges from ADHD they experienced at younger ages don't necessarily go away (especially if they were never addressed). The challenges of ADHD often simply change in terms of how they present (appear) and the problems they create. For example, as children with ADHD move into high school, impulsive behavior often remains an issue even though jumping off the top of monkey bars is no longer the type of problem it causes.

In these years, there are two particularly dangerous aspects to ADHD. One is the risk of abusing drugs and/or alcohol. Once again, there are many theories and explanations as to why there's a greater risk of this in teens with ADHD, from the biological to the psychological to the social. In social terms, teens with ADHD are likely to "hang out" with other underperformers, some of whom may abuse substances, and who collectively reinforce not "buying into" mainstream cultural norms about the value and rewards of dedication, hard work, and achievement. Regardless of arguments about "self-medication" and whatever the short-term effects of a particular substance might be, the regular and repeated abuse of substances inevitably exacerbates challenges with academic performance resulting from the inattentive aspects of ADHD. Substance abuse can also lead to long-term challenges with addiction, as well as the beginnings of what can become a lifetime of trouble with the law.

A second dangerous aspect of ADHD that first becomes an issue at this age involves driving. Both the impulsive and distractible aspects of ADHD can contribute to more than a fair share of vehicle collisions and accidents. This is true in both younger and older drivers. In one study, 6.5% of men and 3.9% of women with ADHD experienced road accidents during a 4-year follow-up period in comparison to 2.6% of men and 1.8% of women without ADHD. In another study that focused on older drivers, there was a 7% increased risk of hard-braking events, a 102% increased risk of self-reported traffic tickets, and a 74% increased risk of self-reported vehicular crashes. This is in fact one of the most serious consequences of untreated ADHD and one that can lead to serious injuries and fatalities (for the person with ADHD, their passengers, and unfortunate bystanders).

The social consequences of ADHD in the teen years are varied, but in general, the social stakes involved with uncontrolled ADHD only get higher and higher as adolescents progress into high school and beyond. A major challenge that often comes up in this age group is that due to inattention, teens with ADHD may miss social cues. Teen society is particularly unforgiving when it comes to sticking to peer norms such as doing and saying the "right" things. Teenagers who don't dress right, don't "stick to the plan," or get a reputation for "blurting things out" are more likely to be ostracized by their peers.

Externally reinforced social exclusion contributes to more voluntary forms of social withdrawal and, in turn, to an increased risk of anxiety and depression.

Finally, a concern about ADHD medications that tends to begin in middle school and high school arises from overlap with anorexia nervosa, a condition in which an individual engages in highly restrictive diets to control their weight. One risk factor for this condition is the misuse of a variety of medications that reduce appetite, including ADHD stimulants. Clinicians treating individuals in this population need to keep their index of suspicion high regarding the risk of disordered eating. It is typically not difficult to separate the two conditions, including by keeping tabs on a teen ADHDer's diet and weight and looking out for potentially problematic behaviors in their eating habits.

College

College raises the stakes to yet another level. In the United States, this is the age when many young adults leave home for the first time for an extended period, during which they are still expected to complete work and perform at a certain level (unlike being at summer camp, by contrast). This is often the first time in an ADHDer's life when they've had the complete lack of an authority figure looking over their shoulder to make sure they do what they need to do, when they need to do it. This naturally can lead to problems keeping up academically, especially for kids whose parents aggressively managed time for them while they lived at home. This setting can also be an issue for a kid with ADHD who got through high school not by systematic hard work but because of natural intelligence (and sometimes by charming their teachers). College may be the first time the challenges from their ADHD become serious enough that they finally seek professional help.

Another social factor that contributes to increasing challenges from ADHD for many college-aged young adults is the normal human desire, which likely began in their teen years, to fit in and not be seen as different. For a young adult with ADHD who has not fully "bought into" either their diagnosis or treatment up to that point, this can often mean that once they leave home, their treatment is not happening anymore. If they were taking medication when at home under pressure from their parents, after they leave they may use the medication only irregularly (for example, to help them stay up all night and "cram" before a test, instead of to keep up with their work and cultivate good study habits) or simply choose not to use it at all.

Sometimes, in fact, the medication begins to serve another social purpose for college students with ADHD: that is, giving away or selling their medication becomes a path to increased popularity and acceptance. Since their parents are no longer able to supervise or monitor the medication, the young adult has freedom to divert the medication toward those who might abuse it (either to cram for tests or to party) or to simply abuse it themselves. Or they may take the money from selling the medicine and use it for something else they prefer to have.

Adulthood

After graduation, people in their 20s are expected to be able to act independently and "stand on their own two feet." But ADHD does not end with the end of school.

Adults with ADHD have some advantages over children with ADHD. For example, adults have more choice than children in how they structure and spend their day. Adults may be able to choose their line of work (and thereby avoid many of the pitfalls of a job that bores them). Depending on the job, no one may care if an employee doesn't keep certain hours so long as they meet certain deadlines. If a worker wants to get all their work done between 2 and 6 in the morning before a major deadline, that might be fine. Adults may also get to decide how messy their desk, office, bedroom, or car is (though this may still cause friction with other people, such as coworkers or those they live with).

That said, being an adult with ADHD is more difficult than being a child with ADHD in many other respects. Due to academic challenges during their school years, some ADHDers start the adult phase of their lives at a disadvantage compared to their peers. They may graduate from high school or college late or not at all, and this has both short- and long-term consequences on their ability to get a job and on their earning potential.

Ironically, given that until relatively recently ADHD was considered a disorder that only affected school-aged children, the consequences of untreated ADHD are often far more severe for adults than for kids. If a child tends to make a lot of silly mistakes in school, the consequence is a poor grade. However, if an adult makes an equivalent mistake at work, such as ordering the wrong item, the whole team or company may be affected by the consequences of the mistake. As a child, if you forgot to do your homework, your parents reminded you until you did it. Your teachers might have docked your grade but might also have let you hand assignments in late and given you a "pass," at least up to a point. But as an adult, the same types of transgressions can get you fired from your job. Once that has happened enough times, it shows up on your résumé and may lead to trouble getting any kind of employment. This of course has huge financial consequences—but the consequences for young adults trying to establish their independence are much more than financial. Not being able to keep a job means not being able to support yourself. It could mean living with your parents or losing your apartment, your car, and other material symbols of your independence. It means increased challenges with dating, finding a lifelong partner, or starting your own family. In short, ADHD in adults presents a huge obstacle to success and self-esteem in addition to increased financial burdens.

Other consequences of ADHD can often be worse in adults than in kids. If your parents got mad at you because you were sloppy as a kid, you likely faced some consequences, but they didn't threaten to put you up for adoption or into foster care. But if your significant other gets frustrated enough, they might leave or divorce you. The government is less forgiving than your grade-school teachers—if you repeatedly forget to file your taxes, you will wind up paying much more in penalties, or might even go to prison. Looking out the side window at a squirrel during class might result in shame when the teacher calls on you and you don't know the answer (or even hear the question). But if you are looking out the side window (or down at your phone) while driving, the consequence could be deadly for you or others. A playground fight might lead to detention. A bar fight or other impulsive, angry outbursts can land you in the hospital with a serious head injury, in jail, or in the morgue—as can substance abuse issues.

As an adult, you don't necessarily have due dates or people telling you what to do or when to do it, but all that unstructured time can open the door to even more significant delays and setbacks. At work, adults with ADHD have difficulties sitting through meetings, paying attention to what is being said, listening to people without interrupting them, prioritizing assignments, and generally remaining productive. And as already emphasized, the challenges from earlier stages of life haven't necessarily gone away. For example, the increased risks of drug and alcohol abuse and of distracted or reckless driving persist.

As an adult living alone, having nobody to remind you to do chores may seem nice until your laundry pile gets so big you can't open a door (or your date mentions the smell—eww!). No one will take your phone away as an adult because you've been on social media for hours. That might seem great at first, but if you don't learn to manage those screen-driven impulses on your own, it will certainly become a curse.

In terms of relationships, ADHD in adults also continues to create challenges. Because of impulse-control issues, adults with ADHD are more likely to enter into poorly considered relationships. Among other downstream problems, this can lead to a greater risk of sexually transmitted diseases and unplanned pregnancies. Adults with

ADHD are also more likely than those without to become victims of domestic violence and abuse. Even with a good partner, challenges the ADHDer has with inattention and distractibility are never a plus when it comes to maintaining a good long-term relationship. "You never listen!" is not a prelude to romance, nor is the constant frustration of "You said you would do this and yet you didn't—again!" The partner of someone with ADHD may resent being put in a position where they feel they have to frequently remind the ADHDer to do their household chores (and then be viewed as a "nag"). Or they may take on more responsibility, believing (often with good reason) that otherwise the job won't get done. Resentment can build on both sides, fracturing the relationship. In a marriage or long-term relationship, in which each partner has to listen to the other and compromise at times, an ADHDer often has a harder time focusing on what their partner says or wants, especially if they are following their own line of thought and haven't bought into their partner's perspective. These and other factors contribute to a higher divorce rate among adults with ADHD. Similar factors also lead to greater rates of depression, anxiety, sleep disorders, and other psychiatric comorbidities in adults with ADHD, as discussed previously in Chapters 4 and 5.

Special Issues When ADHD Adults Become Parents

When adults with ADHD become parents, these issues become magnified, as they become responsible for their children in addition to themselves. Coping with parenthood is stressful enough, but if ADHD has caused issues with holding a job or with relationships, and a child (or two or three . . .) is involved, that can lead to even worse challenges.

> *Tom, 36, was recently diagnosed with ADHD. At the time of his diagnosis, he had two children with his ex-wife and another two with his girlfriend. He had to support all four of them, plus*

> make alimony payments to his ex-wife. He had to coordinate two different school schedules, as the children lived in different school districts. The children did not get along well with each other, contributing to household stress. He had to help manage the transfers back and forth of his two eldest children, as they lived with him part time and his ex-wife part time. The stress of it all contributed to his coping mechanism of internet scrolling, including some soft-porn sites. When his work started to suffer because of this, he was fired. His girlfriend threatened to leave him. He became so depressed he couldn't even face the thought of trying to interview for another job.

Even without the added issues like the ones that Tom faced, raising kids—who may themselves have ADHD, given its heritability—can be more complicated for ADHDers. The organization, emotional control, and listening skills needed to parent a child with ADHD well do not play to an ADHDer's strengths.

ADHD in Pregnant and Breastfeeding Moms

Pregnant and breastfeeding moms have their own specific challenges with ADHD. Most ADHD drugs are rated by the U.S. Food and Drug Administration (FDA) as "Pregnancy Category C," meaning that although there are some studies in animals that demonstrate a risk to the fetus, equivalent studies in pregnant women have never been carried out. To be more specific, there are some reasonable concerns about risk to the developing fetal cardiovascular and nervous systems—although it must be emphasized that no strong causal links have been uncovered. Similarly, many ADHD medications are secreted in breastmilk, at least to some small degree, and so breastfeeding mothers need to take this into consideration before feeding their infants. In some cases it may be possible to minimize transfer to the infant by timing feeds around any stimulant dosing. Infants exposed to stimulants either in utero or via breastmilk are likely to be slightly more irritable and to sleep and feed less until the stimulant leaves their body.

That said, there are certainly risks to both the mother and the fetus from stopping a working ADHD medication. These include re-emergence of the mother's ADHD symptomatology and the related consequences on productivity at home and at work, on self-esteem, and on anxiety. Low self-esteem and high anxiety in the mother are likely to have negative consequences on the baby's development. In a worst-case scenario, these effects can cascade into an increased risk of postpartum depression or even postpartum psychosis in the mother—conditions that can have quite severe and even lethal consequences if left untreated. Unfortunately, this all occurs at a time in the woman's life when focus may be even less sharp: During pregnancy, hormonal changes can contribute to a difference in thinking, which can include worse memory for details and additional attentional issues. And for months after the baby is born (or even longer if the child doesn't sleep well), the sleep deprivation that the mother experiences can also contribute to worse focus, as well as to worse impulsivity, irritability, and emotional dysregulation.

As physicians, we have had numerous patients who decided to keep taking their ADHD medications while pregnant and when breastfeeding (though perhaps at a slightly reduced dose to mitigate such concerns) and who did not have any bad outcomes. While research is still emerging in this area, as a general rule we suggest discussing any treatment decisions with your doctors, and even seeking a second opinion, so you can make a fully informed choice about treatment.

Psychosocial Factors, Part 2: ADHD in the Family

No behavioral disorder exists in isolation. Human beings are social animals, and even as adults, we generally live in families. Moreover, families are often responsible for raising children. Given that it is a behavioral disorder that begins in childhood, ADHD must therefore be discussed in terms of how it impacts families, and how it in turn is impacted by family life.

One big (and obvious) difference between a child and an adult with ADHD is their role in the family. A child's role is generally as a dependent—the expectation is that the child has to do what the adults in the family (and other adults like teachers) want them to do. The adults in the child's life are expected to help the child, including by making decisions for them, whereas the choices of the child are limited.

An ADHD child's experience therefore depends on how their family views their challenges. Different families react in different ways. Some families minimize the issues of ADHD—what may be seen by others as a catastrophic mess may be viewed by this kind of family as a "little bit sloppy." The child is not viewed as problematically hyperactive; rather, they are a bit "spirited" or "energetic." The family does not get concerned until the child has failed multiple classes or has been expelled from school. Some families view this as within the spectrum of normal.

Other families recognize that there are issues but spend a lot of time looking for others to blame: It's the teacher's fault; it's the friend's fault. Sometimes in this situation, parents feel they are protecting their child from the ill will of others. The "mama bear" instinct kicks in, which makes the parent feel good—*I am helping! I am protecting!* However, some "mama bears" can be overprotective to the detriment of their child. By blaming others for their child's issues or always rushing in to help the child, they can make it harder for their child to learn how to help themselves and harder for medical professionals to diagnose and treat their child's ADHD. If a parent is waking their teen in the mornings, sitting with them to make sure they do their homework, and keeping track of their sports equipment for them so they have it for practice, then when the doctor asks, "Are they often late for school? Do they do their homework? Do they lose their belongings?" the answers will not reflect the teen's actual abilities. Because this child can only cope adequately when directly supervised by their parent, that strategy ceases to work once the child leaves the family hearth and has to start making it on their own.

ADHD is hereditary, which means that many children who have ADHD have parents with ADHD. Being a parent in general is hard work—and if both you and your child have ADHD, the work becomes even harder. This is true for all parents, of course, but as mentioned above in the section about sex and gender differences, in most industrialized societies today mothers generally face the greater challenges because in addition to working, they are still often expected to handle the majority of household responsibilities. Taking care of a family means juggling, organizing, and prioritizing a lot of tasks—both their own and those on behalf of the whole family. For a parent with ADHD, let alone a working parent with ADHD, this often becomes impossible. It's difficult to instruct your kids to be better organized when you yourself are not organized or to get them to pay attention or not procrastinate or not leave tasks unfinished when you have the same challenges. The situation for parents struggling with ADHD can wreak havoc with their self-esteem. Continuously hearing "Why can't you just __?" perpetuates and reminds them of their own lifelong struggle with poor performance and the criticism that comes with it.

Another consequence of the hereditary nature of ADHD is that since children with ADHD are more likely to have parents with ADHD, and as adult ADHD is a risk factor for other challenges including divorce, substance abuse, and domestic violence, children with ADHD are more likely to grow up in chaotic family situations, which can further contribute to their behavioral and academic problems.

Parents who have struggled with ADHD themselves often respond emotionally when they see their child struggling with some of the same issues. Sometimes the parent is determined to bend over backward to help their child because they did not feel like they got the help they needed when they were growing up. Other parents have the opposite reaction—*I did it without help, so my child should be able to also!* This can influence how they parent their child, how they interact with their child's teachers, and the decisions they make about their child's diagnosis and treatment, such as whether they are willing to give the child a medication.

Some adults with ADHD may have no financial choice but to extend their time living with their parents or to return to living with their parents after a period of independence followed by unemployment or relationship issues. This is a situation that often contributes to frustration on all sides. It's bad enough struggling with being disorganized and messy, procrastinating, and losing things when you're still a child or when you're an adult living by yourself; it's quite another thing continuing to have those challenges when you're an adult still living under your parents' roof. On the parents' side, these challenges often become a trigger for argument after argument following years of unresolved conflict and struggle.

Children who grow up with untreated ADHD often look back at their childhood and feel they could have done better. Indeed, perhaps the most heartrending aspect of growing up with ADHD is that both as a child and as an adult, no matter how well they perform, the ADHDer frequently thinks, "If they only knew!" They have hidden the disorder, the chaos, and the rush that they always went through to get the job done and feel like an imposter rather than an accomplished person. Decades of struggle with ADHD leads to underperformance and self-blame, as well as to enduring constant criticism from the outside. People grow up thinking they are not smart or not good or that they are always screwing things up. This can often lead to significant problems with depression and anxiety, which create their own issues in family relationships.

Differences in Therapeutic Approaches in Children Versus Adults

In earlier chapters, we discussed treatment for ADHD, including nonmedication and medication approaches. Here, we will briefly point out some differences in treating ADHD in children versus adults.

When it comes to talk-based approaches such as therapy or coaching, there are inevitable differences between what works best for children versus adults. Types of talk therapy that work well for an adult may not be appropriate for a child who hasn't yet developed the necessary abstract reasoning and executive functioning skills needed to make use of it. On the other hand, it is often critical that the families of children with ADHD receive therapeutic assistance in learning how to better cope with and manage the disorder in the child, as well as coaching in how to navigate obtaining educational assistance and accommodations for the child.

In contrast, there are no drug options that work only for children or only for adults. FDA-approved medications for ADHD are identical for adults and children. There are some non–FDA-approved treatments such as antidepressants that are used more in adults and some newer technology-based treatments that have only been proven to work in children so far, but these treatment choices are essentially the same no matter the age of the ADHDer.

That said, depending on the age of the ADHDer, the decision over whether to start a medication often follows different patterns. As a child, you theoretically have some say as to whether to take medication, but practically, there is a lot of pressure to do so if your parents decide you should. Similarly, some teenagers decide they would like to try medication, but their parents don't want them to, or one parent is for it and the other against. This can lead to enormous arguments within a family. In some families where the parents have divorced or separated, the children wind up taking medication at one parent's house and not at the other's.

Adults have more ownership of the decision to take medication. Generally, at the time they decide to take medication, they are in the process of realizing the serious consequences of ADHD on their job or their relationships. They may be worried about potential side effects, but at the point they are considering medication, they tend to recognize that the benefits could be transformational for their lives. Many adults will tolerate side effects when they are the ones taking the medication. But if their kid has side effects, even mild ones, that can raise the parents' hackles and increase their ambivalence about giving the medication to their child, even if they know the same medication helps their own ADHD.

Parents are often more cautious about having their child start taking medication than they are about starting the medication themselves. Parents may worry about whether the medication will negatively affect their child's development, even though generally speaking there no evidence to suggest this. Parents often worry about how long their children will need to be on medication. They sometimes feel guilty about putting their children on medication because they feel they have failed as a parent or are not advocating enough for their child in school. It is all too easy to find horror stories on social media that scare parents, such as those that claim medication can change their child's personality (again, there is little or no evidence to support such claims). Some parents worry that the medications will turn their child into an unfeeling "zombie," and in our experience, even parents of the most hyperactive and difficult children are not looking for zombification!

> Justin, age 7, has already experienced more trouble than many people three times his age. He was kicked out of three preschools before kindergarten. One of the preschools was academically oriented, and his parents agreed it was "not a good fit." However, the other two were play-based preschools, and even there Justin was unable to follow the routines. He was notorious for disrupting circle time, getting into fights on the playground, and taking other kids' toys. When he was asked to leave the third preschool, his parents kept him at home for the 5 months before kindergarten started. For Justin's mom, this meant trying to manage him at the same time she was trying to manage frequent Zoom meetings for her job. Justin wound up in front of screens for hours each day. His mom realized

that this made him even more short-tempered, but she had no choice.

Justin's parents eagerly awaited the start of kindergarten, hoping Justin had matured enough for it. The first month went well, but then old patterns returned. They were called into the school office multiple times—usually it was his mom who attended these meetings, although his dad came to some. The kindergarten teacher was frustrated with Justin. She could tell he could learn, but he was often both disruptive and destructive in class.

By the time first grade came, Justin was already a known "problem child" in his school. He frequently got into trouble, and other kids avoided him. His first-grade teacher expected better self-control than kindergarten level in her pupils, but Justin interrupted and disrupted. He could do his work when he wanted to, but generally he didn't want to.

At this point, Justin's parents spoke with his pediatrician. He was referred to a pediatric neurologist and diagnosed with ADHD. As a first step, the doctor wrote a letter for the school, and the school developed an individualized education program (IEP) for Justin. He was given less work, and the teacher did a positive reinforcement chart for him, where Justin was rewarded with points when he completed work. Although this helped to some degree, problems continued both in class and on the playground. At home, Justin's parents tried to understand the diagnosis and make behavioral modifications with the help of a psychologist.

A few months into second grade, Justin's parents had still not seen much improvement, nor had his teachers. Justin's dad was having trouble sticking to what the psychologist recommended, in part because (as they now realized) he also had ADHD. This caused a lot of marital friction; Justin's mom felt like she always had to play the role of "bad cop" while Justin's dad got to be the "buddy." Justin's academic progress stalled, although all agreed that he could learn easily when he was attentive. Justin's second-grade teacher tried to help, but clearly Justin's work was not at a second-grade level. His art projects stuck out negatively when compared to those of all the other kids. He was below grade level for math and reading. When homework time rolled around each day, he was always too angry to do it—and his mom felt like she was the failure, as she was working from home and nominally in charge of him at homework time. At soccer practices, he would get into fights with his teammates and was asked to leave the team.

At this point, the doctor and Justin's parents had another meeting, and medication was presented as an option. Justin's dad's immediate response was, "No. It's too early. Justin is too young, and he's smart. He'll be OK if we give him more time." But Justin's mom had a different opinion. She felt that Justin was spiraling downward and that she couldn't help him much further. She felt that medication was the best option to normalize his life. Justin's dad remained adamantly against medication—he expressed anger at the doctor, his wife, the psychologist, the teacher, and the school.

This led to heated arguments. Finally, Justin's dad agreed to have him try a medication. Once stabilized on medication, Justin consistently completed his schoolwork. He felt much better about his ability to do his art projects. He became calmer on the playground and started to get invited to birthday parties. He began to make more friends and seemed happier in general. Justin's dad was completely amazed by the transformation he observed in his son. He decided maybe he should finally seek similar help for himself.

Incorporating Differences in ADHD Across the Lifespan into Diagnostic Criteria

When diagnosing ADHD, it's important to consider what is appropriate behaviorally for the age of the person. In other words, symptoms of inattention, impulsivity, or hyperactivity that are abnormal for an eighth grader might be perfectly normal for a fifth grader, whose brain shouldn't be expected to have developed those abilities to the same degree. As doctors, we also have to consider how much a person's family members may be helping them. If a significant other or parent is doing a whole lot of organizing or taking on the person's responsibilities, it can become more difficult to assess the person in question.

Although ADHD is most often a lifelong disorder, the most troublesome symptoms may change over a person's lifetime. The symptoms that you experience as an adult may not be the same exact symptoms that you experienced as a child. For example, as a child you may have lost or misplaced a lot of items, but as an adult, you might not do so because you have learned to be more careful with your items. However, you may have more problems finishing tasks due to distractions as an adult than you did as a child (when life was simpler and when your parents could make you finish things). The fact that ADHD changes over the lifespan is one of the main reasons why the terms "ADD" versus "ADHD" were jettisoned from the DSM-5 in favor of a unified diagnosis—ADHD with different presentations. The idea is that the *presentation* of the disorder can vary over a single person's lifetime (and can also vary in family members with the same genetic predisposition for ADHD), but that the underlying disorder is the same.

Based on the types of symptoms, three presentations of ADHD can occur:

- *Combined: meets both inattentive and hyperactive criteria*
- *Predominantly inattentive: meets only inattentive criteria*

- *Predominantly hyperactive/impulsive: meets only criteria for hyperactive-impulsive*

According to the DSM-5, fewer symptoms are needed to diagnose ADHD in adults than in children. To be diagnosed with ADHD as a child, you must have six or more symptoms in one or both major symptom domains (that is, inattention and hyperactivity/impulsivity), whereas if you're over the age of 17 you only need five or more symptoms total. This is because ADHD can be more difficult to spot in adults than in children. The reasons for this are multifaceted, starting with the fact that ADHD was only relatively recently formalized as a disorder affecting adults—and adults, for all the reasons stated earlier in this chapter, may be more successful at hiding or compensating for the disorder.

To summarize, although the core symptoms of ADHD should be present from childhood, the symptoms of ADHD can change over the lifespan and in different situations. This reflects development of the brain intertwined with familial and social factors—all of which act together to modify the way the disorder presents. Contrary to the long-held view that ADHD is primarily a disorder affecting school-age children, it is now increasingly recognized that the consequences of untreated ADHD can become more serious in adulthood, as adults are held responsible for their actions and their actions have more complex ramifications.

CHAPTER 11

For Care Partners

In this chapter, you will learn:

- What it means to be a care partner
- How to protect yourself when someone else's ADHD affects you
- How to understand and help with the symptoms you can't see as well as the ones you can
- Why caring for yourself is so important
- How to work effectively with your partner's health care team

What Does It Mean to Be a Care Partner?

No one can see ADHD, but it affects a whole lot of people in a whole lot of ways. It affects the actual person with ADHD, of course. But it also affects parents, partners, spouses, siblings, teachers, coaches, therapists, medical professionals, and other caregivers—so this chapter is all about you!

We use the term "care partner" to describe anyone who provides help and support to an ADHDer. The term may make it sound like each person is in the relationship willingly and that the ADHDer is asking for support, but that is not always the case. You might be offering support that your ADHDer does not want. Instead of being grateful for having a partner, the ADHDer may feel like you are trying to boss them around and control them. Rather than getting appreciation, you get resentment. That does not sound much like a "partnership." However, there may be other times when the same ADHDer is grateful for your help and you feel wonderful that you have something important to offer that person. The joy, creativity, and energy of the ADHDer enhances your life when they are at their best.

For parents, teachers, coaches, therapists, and medical professionals, the balance of the partnership is never really equal. In these roles, you generally expect to be doing more giving than getting. It is your job and responsibility to support and guide. However, the ADHDer you are guiding may cause you frustration. You may often find it hard as a caregiver to know how best to react: When confronted by a problem from the ADHDer, you may have a hard time figuring out what behavior is driven by ADHD and what is driven by the person's deliberate choices. Should you get angry? Should you discipline? Or should you be extra-forgiving because, after all, these people have problems that are not their fault?

Society has only recently begun to think about supporting rather than punishing people with ADHD. However, not much attention has been given to the supporters. Parents may feel contradictory and overwhelming emotions: guilt that they are not doing enough, and anger that they are doing so much and it's still not effective. They may spend time feeling anger at their child and the behavior and also anger that other people are not helping their child enough. Spouses may be so frustrated with their partners with ADHD that they frequently yell at them—but still love them. Teachers, coaches, and mental health and medical professionals may feel like they are pouring themselves into helping a person, but in turn the person they are trying to help forgets appointments, doesn't listen, and may not be grateful.

In other words, the spotlight is often on the ADHDer, but the well-being and feelings of the care partners are also important and often overlooked. Many care partners are never asked how they are doing. The care partners may feel selfish or guilt-ridden for having feelings and needs of their own—and every care partner *does* have feelings and needs of their own!

So, let's take some time to think about how care partners can help themselves—seeing as no one else may be doing it.

Acknowledging Feelings and Fears

As mentioned in the preceding paragraphs, it is not uncommon for care partners to have both strong and competing emotions. Here are some common feelings.

Anger

Anger enters relationships with ADHDers in so many ways. It is perfectly natural for care partners to be disappointed and angry with the ADHDer when tasks don't get done properly: "Why can't they just do what they are supposed to?" "How hard is it for them to listen when I talk with them?" "I have asked them a million times, and they just don't seem to care." Parents or significant others may also develop anger toward other care partners who may not be at fault. Parents may fault teachers for not being able to manage their child. Meanwhile, teachers and coaches may blame parents for not disciplining their child enough at home, saying that this has led to their child becoming "unmanageable." Therapists or medical health professionals trying to treat an ADHDer may blame the partners or parents for not being supportive enough—or being too supportive, doing things for the ADHDer rather than letting the ADHDer learn to do it for themselves.

Fear

Your negative feelings may produce innumerable worries and fears, such as:

"Can I trust my ADHD partner to drive safely with the children?"
"What's going to happen if they don't get their act together?"
"Are they going to drop out of school?"
"Are they going to lose their job?"
"How long should I stick it out with this person?"
"How much longer can I last in this relationship?"

Shame

There are many ways that care partners tend to feel ashamed of, or because of, the ADHDer. Shame may come if you are someone who prides yourself on getting to places on time but your ADHD partner makes you constantly late. You may feel that your ADHD partner's lack of organization reflects negatively on you. You may cringe as your ADHD partner acts rudely by interrupting your friends in conversation. And when the teacher of your ADHD child pulls you in to discuss your child's poor grades and "attitude," that certainly does not make you feel proud.

Guilt

Importantly, care partners will often secretly feel guilty for having negative feelings (like the ones just discussed), even when those feelings have been well earned by the ADHDer. For example, a spouse may wonder if they are being unfair for asking their ADHDer to do things they are simply incapable of. This may lead them to doubt the legitimacy of the anger they naturally feel when tasks don't get done properly and to feel guilty about getting angry.

Beyond this, parents tend to feel responsible for the successes and failures of their children. When your child is doing well, whether you truly deserve credit or not, you will often have a lot of good feelings about your parenting. In contrast, when things do not go well for a child with ADHD, parents often fall prey to the notion that they may have somehow failed their child; they feel guilty that they must not be "doing things right." Likewise, teachers, coaches, therapists, and medical professionals may grow frustrated with the lack of success in teaching or treating the ADHDer. They may then wonder if they should be doing something differently and may feel guilty because they don't know how.

> April has been married to an ADHDer, Joe, for 12 years, and they have two children, ages 10 and 6. The 10-year-old also has been diagnosed with ADHD. April loves many aspects of her husband's and child's high energy. "Life is never dull," she says with a chuckle, but she also admits that many aspects of their life are frustrating to her.
>
> When they were dating, one of the things about Joe that attracted April to him was how he was spontaneous and fun-loving. However, as their family and life responsibilities grew, she began to resent that he did not seem to do his fair share of the work. Not only was she the cleaner and finder of things in the house, but Joe seemed to create as much of a mess as the two children combined. She often felt like his butler instead of his wife. She was also constantly apologizing for him to others. For example, he would forget about and miss dinners with friends even when she reminded him that same morning. This was made even worse because Joe was not grateful for the help she often gave him. He would instead get angry with her for "bossing me around." He was still wonderful when it came to things he wanted to do, but they often did not agree on what he should want to do. April came to view Joe as selfish, only participating when he wanted to.
>
> And then they had Charlie, now age 10. Managing Charlie was really difficult for April—and Joe, being "the fun parent," did not really help. In his preschool years, Charlie did not sleep much and needed supervision 24/7. He would bolt across parking lots and climb up and jump off just about anything that was available

to him. When he was 8, while April was inside caring for his younger sister, he pushed the trampoline next to the house to see if he could jump onto the roof. He couldn't, and instead wound up in the ER with a nasty head wound and a disbelieving doctor who was ready to report April to Child Protective Services. She found herself apologizing constantly to other parents when Charlie would be "in the other child's face" or take or break their things. At school conferences she was told, "Charlie is not a good fit for our program." She never knew whether to advocate for him or join others in feeling like he should be punished more. She did not trust him to tell her the truth as he would lie to her about whether or not he had homework. And Charlie mirrored his father in viewing April as a nag: "You're not the boss of me," he would rage.

April did not have much support from anyone. Her parents thought that ADHD was a cop-out and that she and Joe just needed to discipline the child more. Parents of schoolmates who would otherwise have been friendly to her did not want to have her son over. Charlie's soccer coach would constantly bench him for poor behavior during soccer practices, meaning he didn't get the exercise he needed to help dissipate his energy. She was constantly being called by teachers to pick up Charlie from school because "he made poor choices today." On top of everything else, she worried she was neglecting Charlie's sister. Charlie demanded all the energy in the room, in any room he was ever in, and even with all the energy and time April devoted to him, she worried that not only would things not get better, but they would get worse when he became a teenager.

And then, due to his failure to submit his expense reports on time, Joe got laid off from his job. April blamed Joe squarely for that and was angry with him for being so irresponsible. Now, in addition to everything else, the family was being financially squeezed.

There are many "Aprils" out there, and each one of them is dealing with emotions that are not what they envisioned when they "signed up" to be a parent, significant other, teacher, coach, and so forth. They have to reconcile what they hoped would happen in their family with what is actually happening. They have to mourn the loss of the "happy family life" that they had hoped for and cope with the stress of their reality. They have to protect other children from being affected by the tensions created by the behavior of their significant other or child with ADHD.

Care partners like April often feel hesitant to name and express their emotions because they are embarrassed to acknowledge them. It was hard for April to admit that she had really grown to resent Joe when she was so in love with him to begin with. It was hard for April to deal with her son's difficult behaviors when she wanted to love and protect him. As she put it, "It's a slap to my pride when my kid misbehaves." When he got a diagnosis, it alleviated her guilt to some degree but also created new problems. When he misbehaved, she didn't know whether to punish him "for the ADHD, which is not his fault." It took a lot for her to admit that what she had to deal with was more than she could handle on her own.

Sadness. Frustration. Hopelessness. Helplessness. The list of negative emotions that you, like April, may experience as a care partner goes on. And while they may be balanced by love or affection, a sense of responsibility, and other positive emotions, they are still there. It's OK to acknowledge them.

Getting Help

Depression and anxiety are often readily acknowledged in those dealing with a serious medical illness in one they love. For example, if your partner develops cancer, the neighborhood might step in to bring meals to your home, offer you respite and help, and provide you with both physical and emotional support. However, despite the toll it may take on you as the care partner of someone with ADHD, the diagnosis does not routinely trigger similar physical and emotional support from those around you. In fact, you are more likely to be the recipient of negative emotions directed at your loved one with ADHD and at your family.

Here are some ideas that may help you:

1. *Educate yourself about the disorder* (which you are doing by reading this book. Congratulations!). As discussed in Chapter 2, your own vision of ADHD has likely been influenced by society's negative and inaccurate perceptions about the disorder. Luckily, there is now a lot of balanced and helpful information available in books, online, and from local support groups, as well as at conferences you can attend to find out the facts. See Appendix 1, Further Resources, for a list of information. Understanding how your care partner's brain works can be powerful. Knowing that ADHD is no longer considered a disorder caused by "bad kids with bad parents," but instead reflects differences in brain biology, can help alleviate some of the guilt and anger you may be feeling.
2. *Don't dismiss your feelings.* Instead, explore them with other care partners and talk with professionals who are familiar with the issues involved in being a care partner. These discussions should focus on how to support yourself when you're stressed about the ADHDer in your life—they should not be about "how best to support your ADHDer" (there are separate discussions for that). There are parenting coaches, ADHD coaches, and support groups who are there to help you cope for your own sake!
3. *Try to share some of the burden.* Although we acknowledge it may be difficult to find the right people, try to get as much help as you can from doctors, mental health professionals, and others who can help. Don't forget resources in the community such as clergy, athletic coaches, adults whom your child looks up to, and friends who can help you get the jobs done. Don't

forget about outsourcing jobs by using TaskRabbit or similar apps, professional organizers, or cleaners. You don't have to do it all yourself!
4. *If you yourself have ADHD and are not managing it well (remember, it can run in families), consider taking care of your own issues.* (As advised by flight attendants on airplanes, the "put your own oxygen mask on first" method.)

> *April found herself snapping at everyone in frustration with her life spinning out of control. Finally, she decided she needed to get some help. Instead of relying on her husband to pick up their children or to help organize household matters, she hired a college student to work part time in the house. While that put a strain on the family budget, she realized that "it's cheaper than a divorce."*
>
> *She enrolled her son with ADHD in additional after-school sports activities, which gave her a little more time to devote to herself and their other child. She had a few sessions with a therapist who helped her understand she can't be responsible for everything. Just as not everything that went well was her doing, not every problem was her fault, either. If her husband blurted out something rude or her child got into a fight on the playground, that was a reflection on them, not her.*
>
> *While all the problems April had to deal with were still there, getting better at coping with them reduced their impact on her, and she was much happier.*

Focus on the Positives

As discussed in Chapter 7, we all have a **negativity bias** in our brain. That is, the things that go wrong stand out, while our brains often gloss over what is going well. Our brains are built to notice the problems and forget about the victories. As a care partner, this can lead you to become disheartened.

However, there is a solution: You simply have to work harder to notice the positives. It's easy to see when the ADHDer in your life loses an important item or doesn't do a task they were supposed to do. It may be a little harder, but make an effort to notice things they did well. Maybe they got somewhere on time, said something nice to another family member, or took care of a chore. Because of negativity bias, you really have to work to be a balanced observer. The goal should be to recognize three positives for every negative.

Noticing more positives will make you feel happier about your relationship with your loved one who has ADHD. At the same time, the ADHDer will notice you noticing—and be happier with you.

Understand the Invisible Symptoms of ADHD

In some ways, the symptoms of ADHD can seem obvious: forgetting something important, being late, failing to start or finish a task. But as a care partner, you may also be dealing with hidden aspects of ADHD that often go along with these more obvious issues. For example, the ADHDer in your life may be *frustrated with themself* for constantly forgetting things. That frustration often causes more problems than the actual mistake itself, but this frustration may not be visible to you, the care partner. You feel like berating the ADHDer because you have to go all the way back to the restaurant to get the phone that was left behind. You're irritated because you told them to keep it on their lap in the restaurant so they wouldn't forget it. And this is the third time this year (or, possibly, this month!) that this has happened. You are worried about the cost and trouble of replacing the phone if you don't find it.

Meanwhile, the ADHDer is silent and appears not to care. But what is actually going on in their head? They may care deeply about what happened. It's not so much the phone, but what forgetting the phone represents to them. They may be wondering, "What's wrong with me that I keep doing things like this over and over?" They know you are mad at them, and know you have a right to be. They are also mad at themself. They feel foolish or that they've failed—again. These feelings feed symptoms of anxiety and depression. Depression has been described as walking around with an extra-heavy backpack full of misery. People loaded down like that can grow too mentally exhausted to try anymore. The ADHDer may actually be very anxious about what is going to happen without the lost phone. They may worry that even if you do find it, the same thing may just happen again. While the ADHDer may look passive and uninvolved, they may be undergoing significant turmoil inside.

This is often the larger issue. The event will pass—the phone will be found or not. However, the depression and anxiety symptoms the ADHDer is experiencing will linger. And then you, as a care partner, are not dealing with someone who "just" has ADHD. You are dealing with someone who has ADHD, depression, and anxiety, but you are only seeing the ADHD part. The ADHDer may display behaviors that look like irresponsibility, but the larger issue for the mental health of both of you is the hidden anxiety and depression. And that may be harder for you to see when you are angry and frustrated with your ADHDer due to the apparent irresponsibility.

If you work with someone who has had ADHD for a long time, they may have developed coping mechanisms to manage their symptoms. For example, an ADHDer who grew up making lots of silly mistakes may become an adult who copes by double-checking their work a lot. An ADHDer who grew up losing things all the time may become very strict about where they put their keys. An ADHDer who grew up interrupting all the time may be very quiet in group conversations. As their care partner, you may see the double-checking, the care about putting things away, and the quietness. What you may not realize is that those coping mechanisms are super-important to your ADHDer. Trying to get them to change such habits can be very anxiety-provoking for the ADHDer, and they may respond in what you consider an "out of line" way if what you do disrupts or removes their coping mechanism. They may, to you, seem to be ridiculously upset with you if, for example, you move their keys.

No care partner, even those who are the most loving and kind, has psychic powers. The hidden layers of ADHD can silently poison the relationship between you and your loved one with ADHD. Even if you are handling the situation the best you can, you may still have a silently (or sometimes not so silently) upset person in front of you. They may need to calm down before you offer help, give constructive criticism, or even speak with them.

When to Support Versus When to Step Back

How much should you do for the ADHDer in your life? When they are struggling to complete a task, it's often tempting to just step in and do it yourself, whether it's the laundry that is piling up, the room that needs cleaning, the unfinished homework, or the suitcase that needs to be packed for an upcoming trip. Care partners often say, "It's just easier—on everybody—if I do it myself" when, in reality, they actually have mixed feelings about this. Naturally, a common emotion the care partners experience is resentment—Why can't the ADHDer be responsible? Why do I have to do the extra work? Why does everything fall to me?

However, there is also a lot of confusion at play in this situation. For example, the care partner may think:

"Am I doing the ADHDer a disservice by doing this task for them?"
"If I do it, how will they ever take responsibility and learn to do it for themselves?"
"Is it ADHD keeping them from doing the task, or are they just being lazy?"
"Does the ADHDer appreciate me or resent me for helping out too much?"

This is particularly an issue for parents of children with ADHD. It's a central struggle any parent goes through: Should I protect them or let them learn to accomplish things on their own? With the addition of an ADHD diagnosis, the struggle is greater because the parent additionally questions, "How much of this is the ADHD?" Parents often struggle for years trying to figure out which behaviors to excuse. If there are other siblings in the family who don't have these issues, the tendency is to blame the ADHD for every undesirable behavior. But then siblings see the child with ADHD not being disciplined for something they would have been disciplined for! If parents excuse a behavior because of ADHD, how will their child ever learn to behave differently?

The same situation arises when the parent of an ADHDer has to face teachers, administrators, coaches, or other adults when the child is underperforming or causing trouble. Some of these adults may be angry at your child. This tends to arouse a lot of protective instincts in you as the parent. You want to advocate for your child, explaining to the adults why they don't really understand your child or should be easier on them. These instincts can be especially strong during a conference with a teacher about whom your child has been complaining for a long time and who, from the child's perspective, singles them out. You might think the teacher is not making allowances for your child's ADHD. Simultaneously, you might, on some level, also agree with the teacher. You may feel that your child should suffer some sort of negative consequence for the behavior.

Chris was super-mad. He was not sure who he was madder at: his son Steven's high school freshman English teacher, or Steven himself. Steven kept complaining about how the teacher was unfair to him, that she always claimed he talked too much and goofed off in class. Steven was clearly not completing his in-class work, which was the most important contributor to his (poor) grade. His grade was so bad that he would have to go to

> summer school to make it up, ruining the family's plans for a summer vacation. Steven had a 504 plan that was supposed to allow him the accommodation of turning some of his work in late without penalty. However, as part of the 504 plan, he was supposed to ask for that extra time before using it. Chris remembered back to his own youth, when he had to work harder than his peers to keep up because of his own ADHD. In those days, he didn't get a diagnosis, there were no 504 plans, and he was punished by his parents if he did poorly.
>
> In short, Chris was furious with the teacher for not helping his son more, but also furious at his son for not asking for help, for not behaving better in class, and for getting himself into the situation in the first place.

As we've discussed throughout this book, ADHD tends to run in families. If you are biologically related to the ADHDer in your life, there is a higher-than-average chance that you may have the condition as well. That is the case for Chris in the vignette above. He remembers back to when he was a freshman in high school and there were no accommodations for him. He remembers working extra-hard to get his work done and that it took him longer than other kids he knew. He thinks: "I worked hard; why can't he?" His parents would punish him when he did not get his schoolwork done—he remembers being grounded several times for not turning in an assignment on time. He also remembers how it felt to be constantly overworked and criticized while growing up. In fact, he has spent a good part of his adult life getting over his feelings of inadequacy stemming from this personal history. He and his wife have been more accommodating to their son, but Chris is actually not sure whether he should be stricter in this situation. He is constantly hearing from his parents that the only problem with their grandson Steven is that Chris and his wife are too soft on him. Could they be right?

Find Ways to Connect to the ADHDer in Your Life

As we have discussed in the preceding sections, you as a care partner may be experiencing a lot of negative and at times confusing emotions regarding your ADHDer. Navigating these emotions can be difficult. It's therefore important to find some ways to connect with them 100% positively. As a care partner, that will help keep you going!

There are many activities where ADHD is usually not problematic. An ADHDer and their care partner can bond through:

Music—You can either learn an instrument together or just listen to music and talk about it.
Art—Whether it is painting, sculpting, or other media, take a class together or just enjoy! Many communities have "paint night" events you can do together.
Gardening—Adults and children can work together to create a garden, whether it be on a balcony or in a yard.
Sports—Support your local high school or college teams together or splurge on some tickets to see a professional game! You could also play a sport together (pickleball, anyone?) or learn a new one.
Theater—Again, this is something you can go to see. In any community you might find amateurs at all levels or professional shows ranging from basic to elaborate. Or seek out a local theater company that you and your ADHDer can both perform in!
Board games—Pretty much any board game will do! Card games, charades, and other games tend to be a bonding experience, too.
Community service—It's a great experience to work together for the sake of others. Every community has opportunities to serve others: clean up litter, donate to a food bank, or brainstorm your own ways to improve your community. You will develop a sense of shared gratitude for what you have!

These activities act like eyeglasses for you—you can see the ADHDer in a different way. You get to see their creative side, their (good) energy, and their ability to finish what they care about. That is great for the ADHDer; it also helps charge you up so you feel better on days where things don't go so well.

Make Time for Yourself

As already pointed out, flight attendants routinely advise passengers that "you can't help others until you put your own oxygen mask on first." You need "me time" to replenish your emotional tank in order to be able to support your loved one with ADHD. It's not only OK but actually encouraged to take time for yourself. Maybe you could exercise, go for a walk, or go to the beach. Tell everyone you are going out for a while, and if you need to, just take the time to sit and do whatever you want. Which might be nothing!

All of us—including ADHDers and care partners—are at our best when we have plenty of sleep, so be sure to prioritize sleep as part of self-care. Remember, you may need help from others to finish what you started during the day so you can get the sleep you need at night. Lean on your support network as much as necessary. They are out there and there for you!

Summary

Being a care partner is a challenging role, but it can also be incredibly rewarding. Remember that you don't have to go through it alone, and that taking time for yourself is critical. As a care partner, you have needs and feelings too—and those feelings will sometimes be negative and maybe even make you feel guilty or ashamed. We hope we have helped open the door in this chapter for you to connect with others over these important issues, including a local mental health provider for yourself if needed. Please also consult Appendix 1, Further Resources, at the end of this book.

CHAPTER 12

The Gift of ADHD

In this chapter, you will learn:

- What the good sides of having ADHD are

In this book, we have primarily discussed difficulties arising from ADHD. We hope that if you have read this book as an ADHDer (adult or child), or as an ADHD care partner, you now feel better able to manage whatever ADHD throws your way throughout your life!

However, we wish to end this book by re-emphasizing that ADHD isn't all bad: It has its benefits, too. ADHD has aspects you don't have to manage, or cope with, or deal with. ADHD has aspects that bring joy as well. These bear pointing out, as they are easily lost among the more difficult aspects.

For starters, language matters. You can take virtually any ADHD trait and choose to describe it in either a negative or a positive way. For example, "hyperactive" has negative connotations whereas "tireless" is a quality most of us are seeking to achieve. Often at the end of a long week, when a parent is telling us that their child is hyperactive and has too much energy, we find ourselves reflecting that we would like to have some of that energy for ourselves!

The point is to find the right balance when thinking about and describing aspects of ADHD. The natural fountain of energy ADHDers have, once properly focused, includes the ability to blast through any obstacles that come their way. And that can be priceless! Many entrepreneurs with ADHD feel that without the energy they have from their ADHD, and without the sense of inner restlessness carrying them forward to keep doing new things in different ways, they would never have been so successful.

Likewise, there are many contexts in which seeing the big picture "all at once" is more useful than getting bogged down in the details of a particular task. Someone who is too focused may only see "their part" of a project, and that can often be detrimental to success. A basketball player who is too focused on driving down the court themselves may run into a bunch of defenders and never notice the open teammate to whom they could have passed the ball. Similarly, while driving a vehicle, it is important to notice everything around you—if you are only focused on the bit of road directly in front of you, you might miss the car swerving on your right to jump into the lane ahead of you. An ADHDer often has better awareness not just of what is right in front of them, but also of the environment around them, and that can be a gift.

"Be curious, not judgmental" is a quote from Walt Whitman, recently made famous by the TV show *Ted Lasso*. The idea is that in a given situation, it's best to ask questions and learn about what's going on rather than to quickly judge. We feel this phrase is also applicable to ADHDers, who as a whole tend to be very curious about a lot of things. Part of the reason is that ADHD leads them to notice lots of little details that other people don't. The downside is that sometimes this can interfere with identifying what is most important in the current situation, but there is a major upside to seeing things that other people miss.

Possibly because they are less likely to get "hung up" on extraneous details in their heads, ADHDers may sometimes have quicker reaction times. This is often a benefit in sports and could be part of the reason why more athletes have ADHD than the general population. The impulsiveness of ADHD can also translate into a greater flexibility to abandon a plan if something better occurs to them. The ADHDer's lack of inhibition can help them do (really scary, to some of us) sports such as extreme skiing, wingsuit flying, or parkour. While being a successful athlete certainly requires focus and discipline, if the ADHDer enjoys a sport, their distractibility will go down and the benefits of speed and flexible reaction times can really let them shine.

Even for non-athletes, willingness to take risks can confer a huge benefit in many aspects of life. It's a necessity for anyone who starts a company. If you are going to try doing anything new, you have to be able to take the risk that it may not work out—and that is something that many ADHDers are comfortable with. Part of the reason for this is that ADHDers have often lived their lives trying to do things "outside the lines" without guaranteed success; they accordingly grow willing to take risks that most ordinary people without ADHD would never consider.

ADHDers also do well in situations that garner immediate results. They tend to gravitate toward results-oriented fields of work in which they are rewarded early and frequently. Often this can come in the form of work in which moving around a lot or moving from task to task quickly is rewarded. Examples include working in sales, working as a line chef, firefighting (literally putting out fires), or working in information technology/customer support (putting out figurative fires).

Finally, ADHD also may come with the ability to think more creatively. ADHDers tend to be not just good but great at generating many different ideas from a single starting point (this is called divergent thinking). This means that ADHDers are much better than average at looking at a problem and finding new solutions for it. They are also great at thinking of completely different ways to use the same object—for example, using a chopstick not just for eating but also for staking plants in the garden (this ability is called conceptual expansion). As a result of these strengths, ADHDers are also good at moving past old or established thinking. For example, if asked to invent something, they tend to come up with something unique rather than just improving an old product. If asked to imagine what life is like on an alien planet, they don't just come up with variations of what we have on Earth; they imagine completely different life forms or the foods those life forms might eat. Generally, drawings by ADHDers tend to be rated higher in terms of creativity and originality. This "outside the box" style of thought is a skill that people without ADHD try to learn to give them an edge in fields requiring innovation and creativity, but it's something that ADHDers are naturally good at!

We hope this book will help remind you, either as an ADHDer or as a person caring for an ADHDer, that the disorder comes with positives as well as negatives. The strategies in this book and resources presented in Appendix 1, Further Resources, can help you minimize the downsides of ADHD while playing to its strengths, leading to greater mental well-being and success.

GLOSSARY

504 plan: Section 504 of the Rehabilitation Act of 1973 prohibits discrimination on the basis of disability in programs or activities that receive federal financial assistance from the U.S. Department of Education (that is, all public schools).

A

Accommodation: A modification to an educational or work environment that allows an individual with a recognized disability to gain access to assigned content or to complete tasks.

ADD: See Attention-deficit Disorder, below.

ADHD coach: A professional dedicated to helping clients learn how to better manage and cope with the challenges (and maximize the benefits) of ADHD.

ADHDer: Someone who has ADHD.

Adrenaline (aka epinephrine): A chemical released in the body in response to stress. Adrenaline increases heart rate, blood pressure, and perspiration and dilates the pupils to help the body respond to stress or a threat (the "fight-or-flight response"). When disordered this reaction can also lead to a panic attack. Chemically, adrenaline/epinephrine is closely related to noradrenaline/norepinephrine, a neurotransmitter affected by ADHD.

Affect (noun): The facial expression of emotions.

Affective reactivity/lability/dysregulation: Rapidly changing or unstable emotional expression.

Agoraphobia: Fear of leaving one's home; often a consequence of extreme generalized anxiety or panic disorder.

Allele: A difference in the instructions for one gene, often consisting of a change in a single "letter" of the genetic code (an "A" instead of a "C," for example) in just one place.

Amygdala: An almond-sized brain region that is part of the **limbic system** or **salience network**, involved in detecting and responding to fear, threats, and other types of negative stimuli and emotions.

Angular gyrus: A region of the parietal lobe immediately adjacent to the temporal lobe and involved in processing complex language functions; a component of the **default mode network**.

Anterior cingulate cortex: A region of the brain located near the front-center—resembling a "collar" around the front of the **corpus collosum**. Involved in attention allocation, reward anticipation, decision-making, impulse control, performance monitoring, error detection, and emotion.

Antidepressant: A medication used to treat symptoms of depression.

Anxiety: A clinical term for excessive worrying, rumination on negative thoughts, or fear. There are a range of anxiety disorders defined in the **DSM**, including **generalized anxiety disorder, panic disorder, post-traumatic stress disorder**, phobias, and more. Anxiety can interfere with concentration and cause agitation, which can mimic or exacerbate ADHD (see **diagnostic mimicry**).

Arsenic: A metalloid element (atomic number 33) that is toxic to the central nervous system.

Attention-deficit disorder (ADD): An outdated term for ADHD with predominantly inattentive presentation.

Attention-deficit/hyperactivity disorder (ADHD): The current term for a neuropsychiatric condition characterized by symptoms related to one or more of three behavioral domains: inattention, hyperactivity, and impulsivity. Some people with ADHD have symptoms mostly in just one domain, while others have symptoms in a combination of two or all three domains. These combinations are referred to as different **presentations** of ADHD.

Attention network: See **central executive network** and **DMN interference model**.

Autism spectrum disorder (ASD): A developmental condition existing in a wide range of severity, with aspects such as challenges with social interactions and communication, limited interests, or repetitive behavior. Autistic people frequently have differences in their ability to pay attention or in their movements that can cause ASD to be confused with ADHD.

B

Basal ganglia: A network of small interconnected brain regions located near the center on both the right and left sides. The basal ganglia are involved in the execution of voluntary movement, processing sensory and emotional information, and evaluating potential reward and risk. They are anatomically closely associated with the directly adjacent **limbic system**.

Bioenvironmental correlation: The notion that biological and environment factors (such as those contributing to ADHD) do not occur independently but are often linked together. This link can make it difficult to determine causation in epidemiological studies (that is, was something caused by biology, the environment, or both?).

Biology: The branch of science focused on all living things. Mechanistically speaking, it is the study of the ways living things operate at all levels (molecularly, chemically, physiologically, interactively, and more).

Biomarker: A biological finding or characteristic that can be assessed as part of a medical test, usually to help in making a definitive diagnosis.

Bipolar disorder: A psychiatric disorder characterized by "mood swings." A person with bipolar disorder may be depressed at some times but have mania or hypomania (that is, have lots of energy and be abnormally upbeat or irritable) at others. Both depression and mania/hypomania can sometimes mimic or exacerbate aspects of ADHD.

Blood test: A test for biomarkers in the blood.

Brain circuits/networks: Connections between different brain areas.

Brain-derived neurotrophic factor (BDNF): A protein produced in the brain that plays an important role in brain cell survival and growth, serves as a neurotransmitter modulator, and participates in brain plasticity essential for learning and memory.

Brain scan: An imaging test of the brain.

C

Cannabis: Marijuana

Cardiology/cardiologist: The branch of medicine (or a physician) specialized in disorders of the heart.

Care partner: Anyone who provides support to an ADHDer.

Caudate: A small brain region forming part of the **basal ganglia** that helps in planning voluntary movement and processing many other types of information.

Causal: Relating to or acting as a cause.

Central executive network (CEN): See **DMN interference model**.

Cerebral cortex: The outermost layers of the main part of the human brain (cerebrum); the part most expanded in humans relative to other animals.

Cerebral palsy: A condition marked by impaired muscle coordination and/or other disabilities, typically caused by damage to the brain before or during birth.

Child neurologist/child psychiatrist: A neurologic or psychiatric specialist who focuses specifically on disorders of children (vs. those of adults).

Coach/Coaching: A form of support for ADHD and/or ADHD caregivers focused on teaching practical coping strategies to better manage and control challenges presented by the disorder. Can overlap substantially with "Therapy/Therapist" (see below), but distinct in part for historical reasons.

Cognitive behavioral therapy (CBT): A type of talk therapy focused on training in skills to identify and change one's habits of thought (cognition) and action (behavior), with the goal to mitigate symptoms and/or cope with challenges created by a mental health condition.

Comorbid (adjective); comorbidity (noun): Refers to two or more medical conditions occurring together in the same patient. Many psychiatric conditions, including ADHD, have high rates of comorbidity with other psychiatric conditions (for example, ADHD and depression).

Computed tomography (CT) scan: A type of imaging technique in which a computer is used to piece together a 3D image of an organ using a high number of sequential 2D X-ray images. When used to assess the brain, a CT scan can reveal the anatomy (structure) of different brain regions (though not their activity).

Continuous Performance Task/Test: A computerized test of attention/impulsivity in which a user is asked to sit still and perform a simple repetitive task for 15–20 minutes. It is scored based on normal population data.

Corpus callosum: A tract of fibers connecting the left and right hemispheres of the brain that facilitates long-distance and bilateral communication between many brain regions.

Correlational: In terms of study design, a type of research study in which one factor is correlated with another in hopes of identifying a possible causal relationship. However, a frequently quoted truth is that "correlation does not equal causation." In other words, just because two things tend to occur together does not prove that one caused the other.

Cycle of failure: A vicious cycle of behavior, all too common in those with ADHD, in which a history of not meeting goals or expectations contributes to low self-esteem, decreased motivation, and hopelessness, which in turn can lead to procrastination, poor effort, and giving up easily in the face of challenges. The cycle of failure in ADHD increases the likelihood of further failures in meeting goals and expectations.

Cycle of success: A virtuous cycle of behavior. As applied to ADHD it refers to setting attainable goals and celebrating each accomplishment, which leads to increased self-esteem and motivation to apply oneself, a greater ability to overcome obstacles, and the ability to set increasingly ambitious goals over time.

D

Default mode network (DMN): See **DMN interference model**.

Depression (see also major depressive disorder, major depressive episode): A psychiatric disorder characterized by excessively low mood that can also interfere with motivation, energy levels, sleep, appetite, and concentration (and that is therefore often confused with, or can contribute to, symptoms of ADHD).

Developmental delay: A condition in which a child or adult has abnormally low mental ability for their age.

Diabetes: A medical condition in which the pancreas does not secrete enough insulin, leading to abnormally high blood sugar levels. It can result from long-term poor eating habits.

Diagnostic and Statistical Manual of Mental Disorders, Fifth Edition (DSM-5): The official classification system of mental disorders created and periodically revised by the American Psychiatric Association. This manual is used by psychiatrists and other medical professionals in the United States. It is also influential in other parts of the world and has influenced diagnostic systems such as the International Classification of Diseases (ICD), created and periodically revised by the World Health Organization.

Diagnostic mimicry: The idea that one medical or psychiatric diagnosis can mimic another. A significant part of both the "science" and "art" of medicine and psychiatry involves learning how to differentiate between such diagnoses. In the case of ADHD, there are many other psychiatric and medical conditions that can "masquerade" as ADHD or contribute to its severity. Conversely, untreated ADHD is often mistaken for (or contributes to) other diagnoses such as depression and anxiety.

Dialectical behavioral therapy (DBT): A form of therapy that draws on cognitive behavioral therapy, mindfulness techniques, and philosophical traditions to help a person better understand, process, and control automatic or habitual negative mental, emotional, and behavioral responses; to foster acceptance; and to improve interpersonal relationships.

Dissociation: A state in which a person loses touch with reality—for example, feeling that the world around them isn't "real" or that they are outside their own body. It can be a reaction to extreme anxiety.

DMN interference model: One hypothesis that seeks to explain ADHD based on current understanding of brain networks. The idea is that a network of brain regions normally active when the brain is not focused (the default mode network [DMN]) is overconnected to a different network that is normally active when the brain is focused (the task positive network [TPN], aka the central executive network [CEN]).

Dopamine: A neurotransmitter implicated in ADHD because of its effects on cognition, sensory processing, and attention (but also involved in reward, movement, psychosis, and lactation).

Dopamine transporter (DAT) scan: An experimental brain scan that uses a radioactive compound to detect brain areas that are actively using dopamine.

Dorsomedial prefrontal cortex: A subdivision of the prefrontal cortex, arrayed along the front midline of the brain—a component of the default mode network.

Dyslexia: A specific learning disability that affects how the brain processes and decodes written language.

E

Educational Psychology/Psychologist: A psychologist who specializes in assessing students for learning disabilities, often as part of the process of developing a 504 Plan or IEP.

Electroencephalogram (EEG): A recording of brain waves made by placing leads on a person's scalp and comparing electrical potentials across them. Brain waves are a crude but clinically useful measure of overall activity across different regions of the brain. They vary in different states of consciousness and sleep and are abnormal during an epileptic seizure. They cannot be used to measure cognitive features such as someone's thoughts or emotions or to independently diagnose a psychiatric condition. See neuropsychiatric EEG-based assessment aid (NEBA) system to learn about their use in the diagnosis of ADHD.

Elimination Diet: Any one of several diets designed to eradicate the ingestion of supposed toxins or allergins believed to contribute to a disorder such as ADHD.

Enzyme: A naturally occurring protein that catalyzes (promotes) a specific chemical reaction in the body.

Epidemiology/Epidemiological: Relating to the branch of medicine that deals with the incidence, distribution, and control of diseases.

Epilepsy: A neurologic disorder marked by recurrent episodes of convulsions, sensory disturbances, or loss of consciousness associated with abnormal electrical activity in the brain. May also be called a seizure disorder.

Executive functioning: The use of working memory, impulse inhibition, balance between risk versus reward, and reasoning to organize tasks, manage time, plan, and solve problems.

F

Family medicine: A branch of primary care that focuses on the prevention, diagnosis, and care of basic health issues in both children and adults.

Frontal lobe: One of the major subdivisions of the human brain, located on either side directly behind the eyes and forehead.

G

Gene: The instructions encoded in DNA to make a single building block of a living being—generally speaking, one protein. The complete set of instructions to make a human being is encoded by approximately 25,000 genes (modulated by a lot of other DNA regions that are not considered genes).

Generalized anxiety disorder: A psychiatric condition characterized by excessive worrying, intrusive negative thoughts, or fears about a range of different things. Common symptoms are insomnia, loss of appetite, and abnormal or uncomfortable body sensations and symptoms (such as headaches, dizziness, stomach pains, diarrhea or constipation, nausea, tingling limbs, or tinnitus). In extreme cases, this may be accompanied by **panic attacks**, **agoraphobia**, or **dissociation**.

Genetic tests: Testing for diagnosis of a medical condition (or for assessing metabolism or responsiveness to different drug types) by sequencing or otherwise examining a person's genes—in other words, looking for genetic variations associated with disease.

Geriatric Medicine/Provider: The branch of medicine focused on the diagnosis, prevention, and treatment of diseases in the elderly.

H

Heart disease: Any disease of the heart. Sometimes used conventionally for cardiovascular disease resulting from poorly controlled cholesterol levels and/or high blood pressure, which make a person prone to heart attacks and strokes.

Heavy metals: A metal of high atomic density, such as aluminum, arsenic, cadmium, lead, or mercury, exposure to which can damage the brain.

Heritability: The proportion of variation in a trait attributable to genetic factors. In terms of ADHD, this means the proportion of ADHD risk that comes from differences between people's DNA versus other influences such as environmental factors.

Hippocampus: A component of the **limbic system** involved in learning and memory; also often considered a part of the **default mode network**.

Hyperactive/hyperactivity: Excessive movement, fidgetiness, or the inability to sit still. Part of the behavioral triad of ADHD (inattention, impulsivity, and hyperactivity).

Hyperfocus: The concept that some people, including some people with ADHD, are prone to focusing on a single task, often to the exclusion of everything else and sometimes in a maladaptive fashion.

Hyperkinetic: Another term for hyperactive.

Hypomania: A mood state characterized by euphoria and/or irritability, high levels of energy, reduced need for sleep, pressured speech, distractibility, impulsivity, and poor judgment. A characteristic of **bipolar disorder**.

I

Impulsivity: Difficulty controlling one's behavior and considering consequences before taking an action. Another part of the behavioral triad of ADHD (inattention, impulsivity, and hyperactivity).

Inattentiveness: Difficulty focusing on a task or the speech of another person; distractibility. One part of the behavioral triad of ADHD (inattention, impulsivity, and hyperactivity).

Individualized education program (IEP): A written plan for a child with an identified disability describing how to approach their education and provide resources to accommodate the child's challenges in school and help the child overcome them. Developed through collaboration between teachers, school counselors, parents, the child, and the child's clinical providers, including pediatricians, psychologists, neurologists, and psychiatrists.

Insomnia: The inability to fall asleep, stay asleep, or get adequate sleep.

Internal medicine/internist: The branch of medicine that focuses on diagnosis, prevention, and treatment of diseases in adults.

In utero: Inside the womb (that is, during embryonic and fetal development, before a baby is born).

L

Lead exposure: See heavy metals.

Limbic system: A network of small brain regions located near the center on the right and left sides. It is involved in positive and negative reinforcement (for example, reward/risk/punishment) and associated emotions (for example, pleasure, satisfaction, happiness, fear, revulsion, hatred) as well as critical survival behaviors (for example, feeding, sex, nursing, and fight-or-flight responses). It is anatomically closely associated with the directly adjacent basal ganglia.

Locus (plural: loci): A defined segment of a DNA molecule. Not every locus corresponds to a gene. In fact, most of your DNA isn't genes—instead, it's regulating where/when genes are turned on and off.

M

Magnetic resonance imaging (MRI) scan: A technique in which a 3D image is taken using high-intensity electromagnets to detect differences in a structure's internal water density. As applied to the brain, an MRI scan, like a CT scan, can reveal brain anatomy (structure) but not activity.

Major depressive disorder/major depressive episode (see also Depression): A psychiatric condition in which an individual has a debilitating low mood for 2 weeks or longer. Other symptoms may include reduced ability to experience pleasure, suicidal thinking, low energy, poor motivation, difficulty thinking and concentrating, sleeping too much or too little, and disordered eating. A person may experience a major depressive episode only once in their life or may experience repeated or chronic episodes (that is, recurrent major depressive disorder).

Mania (see also Hypomania): A more extreme version of hypomania. A mood state characterized by euphoria and/or irritability, high levels of energy, reduced need for sleep, pressured speech, distractibility, impulsivity, poor judgment, and a marked deterioration in functioning that can include delusional and/or paranoid thought patterns. Characteristic of **bipolar disorder**.

Mental Status Exam: A standardized summary of a patient's mental state as viewed by their doctor. The equivalent of a physical exam for psychiatry and psychology.

Mercury: See **heavy metals**.

Monoamine: A class of neurotransmitter characterized by having a single nitrogen (a "monoamine" group) as part of their chemical structure. There are three closely related major monoamines in the human brain: serotonin (psychiatrically implicated in depression and anxiety), dopamine (implicated in depression, psychosis, addiction, and ADHD), and norepinephrine (implicated in depression, anxiety, and ADHD).

Mood Disorder: A mental disorder in which the primary symptom is a disruption of mood—major depression, bipolar disorder, etc.

Myelination (myelinating): A normal process during brain development that involves laying down a fatty insulating layer around nerve fibers; this contributes to faster, more efficient communication between brain cells connected at a distance by these fibers.

N

National Institutes of Health (NIH): A federal agency that oversees medical research in the United States; one part of the U.S. Department of Health and Human Services.

Negativity bias: A natural bias that leads to negative events having a greater effect on a person's psychological state than those that are neutral or positive.

Neurodevelopmental: Corresponding to the process of brain growth—that is, the natural process by which the nervous system develops both before and after birth.

Neurodevelopmental disorder: Any medical condition thought to result from an irregularity that occurred during brain growth.

Neurology/Neurologist: The branch of medicine (or a physician) focused on disorders of the human central nervous system; one of the three types of medical specialists focused on the brain (the others being **psychiatrists** and neurosurgeons). Neurologists typically treat patients by prescribing medications.

Neuron: One of the primary cell types in the brain, whose electrochemical activities and communications underlie all mental functions.

Neuropsychiatric EEG-based assessment aid (NEBA) system: A brain wave test approved by the U.S. Food and Drug Administration (FDA) that can be used to assist (along with other aspects of a proper neuropsychiatric evaluation) in the diagnosis of ADHD.

Neuropsychiatry/neuropsychiatric: An umbrella term for disorders of the brain that affect emotions and behavior and that therefore could be treated either by neurologists or psychiatrists. To some degree, all neurologic and psychiatric disorders are "neuropsychiatric," since the division between neurology and psychiatry is mostly historical and practical, as opposed to biological or scientific.

Neuropsychological testing: Exams given by a trained psychologist designed to measure a range of mental abilities. This can include aspects of ADHD, such as attention, but typically also includes many other cognitive abilities such as reading and mathematical ability, visuospatial processing, and memory.

Neurotransmitter: A naturally occurring chemical in the brain that is released between neurons (at synapses), allowing them to signal to each other.

Neurotransmitter receptor: A protein on the receiving end of the synapse that governs the response of the receiving neuron to a particular neurotransmitter signal.

Norepinephrine (noradrenaline): A neurotransmitter implicated in ADHD because of its effects on alertness, but also involved in both depression and anxiety. Released primarily in the brain, it is a close chemical analog of epinephrine/adrenaline.

Nucleus accumbens: A brain region that is part of the **limbic system**, involved in motivation and reward.

Nurse Practitioner (NP): A nurse who has received specialized training allowing them to diagnose and treat certain patients either on their own or under the supervision of a physician.

O

Obsessive-compulsive disorder (OCD): A psychiatric disorder characterized by the repeated experience of unwanted thoughts and fears (obsessions) that can lead to the performance of repetitive and ritual-like behaviors (compulsions).

Obstructive Sleep Apnea : A medical condition in which a physically compromised airway leads to disrupted sleep at night, leading to poor sleep quality and a range of psychological and medical consequences (including attentional difficulties).

P

Paleogenetics: The analysis of DNA sequences from prehistoric samples—for example, from the bones of ancient human ancestors.

Panic attack/panic disorder: A severe anxiety disorder characterized by physical symptoms often including tightness in the chest, high heart rate, heart palpitations, shortness of breath, perspiration, tingling or pain in the limbs, feelings of paralysis, muscle jerking, a narrowing or darkening field of vision, and overwhelming feelings of dread ("the world is about to end" or "I'm going to die"). A panic attack may be mistaken for a heart attack and result in an ER visit, especially the first time one occurs.

Parent–child interaction therapy: A form of therapy developed by child psychologists and child psychiatrists, designed to analyze the behavioral and verbal dynamics between children and their parents during play or task completion and to provide strategies for improving such interactions.

Parent management training: A form of therapy or coaching focused on helping parents learn techniques to more productively interact with their children who are having attentional, impulse control, or other behavioral issues.

Parietal lobe: One of the major subdivisions of the human brain, located on either side, behind the frontal lobes and above the temporal lobes.

Pathological: Corresponding to a medical disease or condition—used to describe a biological or mental process or behavior that contributes to a medical illness. Note that when it comes to the human mind and behavior, there is wide variation around what is "normal." Only when a mental process or behavior is so extreme as to cause significant problems in function is it considered "pathological."

Pediatrics/pediatrician: The branch of medicine (or a physician) focused on the diagnosis, prevention, and treatment of diseases in children.

Penetrance: In genetics, the degree to which an **allele** causes a predictable change in an organism (like a human being). Many alleles are not 100% penetrant. With regard to ADHD, for example, even if you have an allele that contributes to ADHD in somebody else (say, your own identical twin), that doesn't predict with 100% certainty that it will cause you to have ADHD as well.

Play therapy: A form of therapy developed by child psychologists and child psychiatrists designed to help young children, who may not yet have developed the words or modes of abstract thought to fully express themselves verbally. In this type of therapy, the child expresses and processes their feelings through interactive play.

PMHNP: See Psychiatric and mental health nurse practitioner, below

Positron emission tomography (PET) scan: A type of imaging technique in which a computer is used to piece together a 3D image of an organ by detecting positrons emitted from a radioactive tracer. As applied to the brain, a PET scan provides less detailed anatomy than a CT or MRI scan, but it can indirectly detect the relative activity in different brain regions (by imaging blood flow or glucose use, for example).

Posterior cingulate cortex (precuneus): A subregion of the cingulate cortex located immediately behind the **anterior cingulate cortex**, near the center of the brain. A component of the **default mode network**.

Post-traumatic stress disorder: A psychiatric diagnosis that originally grew out of the study of "shell shock" in military veterans after WWI. It is now recognized to occur in many people, including civilians, who have been exposed to an extreme acute threat (or, as is now increasingly being recognized, a more chronic low level of threat, such as that occurring in an emotionally abusive household).

Precuneus: See **posterior cingulate cortex**.

Prefrontal cortex: The outermost layer of the foremost part of the frontal lobes of the brain, located right behind the eyes and forehead. This is the brain area most uniquely expanded in modern humans compared to other animals. It functions in decision-making.

Presentation: A medical term for how a disease or disorder appears in a patient, especially as first seen in a doctor's office.

Prevalence: How common a medical condition is at any given point in time, expressed as a percentage of the total population.

Psychiatric and mental health nurse practitioner (PMHNP): A nurse practitioner who has received specific training and certification in the diagnosis and treatment of mental health conditions.

Psychiatry/psychiatrist: The branch of medicine (or a physician) focused on the human mind or psyche; one of three types of medical specialists focused on disorders of the brain (the others being **neurologists** and neurosurgeons). Psychiatrists typically treat patients by prescribing medications, though they may also use talk therapy or other types of non-medication approaches.

Psychoactive Drug: Any drug, whether taken with a prescription or not, that affects the mind, mood, or consciousness.

Psychoanalysis: A type of therapy, first developed by Dr. Sigmund Freud in the late 1800s and early 1900s, focused on identifying and exposing unconscious fears and conflicts and bringing them to consciousness through techniques such as dream interpretation and free association. (Not recommended as a specific treatment for ADHD.)

Psychology/psychologist: The branch of science (or a practitioner) concerned with the emotions, thoughts, and behaviors of human beings and other sentient species. Psychologists are professionals who either research behavior or treat it in humans, generally without using medications (that is, via talk therapy or behavioral interventions).

Psychosis: A condition in which a person experiences hallucinations (abnormal or incorrect sensory perceptions) and/or delusions (bizarre thoughts and/or incorrect explanations for why things are happening), including paranoia. Psychosis is a primary symptom of schizophrenia but can also be present in bipolar disorder, severe depression, or as a result of substance abuse or a medical condition.

Putamen: A brain region forming part of the **basal ganglia** that helps in the preparation and execution of movement, including speech; also involved in some aspects of learning and reward.

Q

Qualitative: Relating to or measured by the quality, type, or kind of something rather than by its quantity or degree.

Quantitative: Relating to or measured by the quantity or degree of something, rather than by its type, kind, or quality.

R

Radiolabelled tracer: A chemical, either ingested or injected into the bloodstream, that (by virtue of being radioactive) is visible on a scan and thereby facilitates visualization of a specific target.

Recall bias: A psychological phenomenon in which a human being tends to remember events differently from the way they actually happened or with a skew—see also "negativity bias".

Retrospective: A type of clinical study in which a correlation is sought between some present outcome and events that took place in the past.

S

Salience network: See **triple network model**.

Schizophrenia: A mental disorder that is characterized by **psychosis** and that often includes symptoms overlapping with other neuropsychiatric disorders, including low mood, lack of facial expression, odd movements, low motivation, poor concentration, and attentional difficulties.

Seizure disorder: See **epilepsy**.

Single photon emission computed tomography (SPECT) scan: A type of imaging technique in which a computer is used to piece together a 3D image of an organ by detecting gamma rays emitted by a radioactive tracer. As applied to the brain, a SPECT scan provides less detailed anatomy than a CT or MRI scan but can indirectly detect the relative activity in different brain regions by imaging blood flow.

STD: Sexually transmitted disease.

Synapse: A specialized junction between neurons (brain cells) where they communicate through the rapid release and reception of chemical signals (**neurotransmitters**).

T

Talk therapy: See "therapy/therapist".

Task positive network (TPN): See **DMN interference model**.

Temporal lobe/temporal cortex: One of the major subdivisions of the human brain, located on either side roughly below the temples.

THC: Tetrahydrocannabinol: The main psychoactive compound (drug) found in marijuana.

Therapy/Therapist: Any one of several types of professionals dedicated to helping clients overcome mental health challenges by talking to them. Goals are generally to increase insight into cognitive, emotional, and behavioral challenges, identify the psychological sources of these challenges, and learn practical coping strategies to better manage and control them.

Tolerance: A diminished response to a drug that occurs when the drug is used repeatedly, leading to a need for higher doses to generate the same effect. In contrast to drugs like opioids, which are highly prone to tolerance and resultant abuse, prescription stimulants typically have a more limited capacity to generate tolerance.

Transcranial magnetic stimulation (TMS): A treatment for brain disorders that uses a fluctuating magnetic field generated by an electromagnet to either increase or diminish the activity of targeted brain circuits. (Not currently approved by the U.S. Food and Drug Administration [FDA] for ADHD.)

Trigeminal nerve stimulation (TNS): A treatment that has been approved by the U.S. Food and Drug Administration (FDA) for ADHD in children that uses non-painful, low-level superficial stimulation of one of the upper facial nerves during sleep to modulate brain circuits involved in ADHD, particularly executive functioning.

Triple network model: A slightly more complex or sophisticated version of the **DMN interference model** of ADHD that incorporates a third brain network. According to this model, the **salience network (SN)**, involved in noticing when something in the environment is worth paying attention to, helps coordinate negative anticorrelation (that is, reciprocal activity or "switching") between the DMN and TPN.

U

Urology/Urologist: The branch of medicine (or a physician) specialized in disorders of the kidney and associated urinary organs.

V

Variant: A difference in the genetic code at a particular **locus**. Variants range in how common they are in the human population. Some are associated with an increased risk for a disease or psychiatric disorder (like ADHD), others contribute to non-medical trait differences (such as height or hair or eye color), and many are silent (do nothing). The term is generally used to mean a difference in DNA that has been inherited, as opposed to a de novo genetic difference (mutation) occurring in just one individual.

Vicious cycle: A negative feedback loop—that is, one bad thing causes a second bad thing, which then "feeds back" to reinforce or increase the first bad thing again, and so on. As applied to ADHD, a history of not meeting goals or expectations contributes to low self-esteem, decreased motivation, and hopelessness, which in turn leads to procrastination, poor effort, and giving up easily in the face of challenges. See also **cycle of failure**.

Virtuous cycle: The opposite of a **vicious cycle**. A virtuous cycle is a positive feedback loop where the consequences are increasingly good instead of increasingly bad. For instance, regular cardiovascular exercise leads to being in better physical shape, which leads to having more energy to continue to exercise regularly, and so on. As applied to ADHD, the virtuous cycle refers to setting attainable goals and celebrating each accomplishment, which leads to increased self-esteem and motivation to apply oneself, a greater ability to overcome obstacles, and the ability to set increasingly ambitious goals over time. See also **cycle of success**.

APPENDIX 1

Further Resources

Informational Websites

ADDitude Magazine: https://www.additudemag.com/
ADD WareHouse: ADD WareHouse has the largest collection of ADHD-related books, videos, training programs, games, and assessment products in the world. www.addwarehouse.com
Attention Deficit Disorder Association (ADDA): The ADDA's mission is to work with adults who have ADHD to lead better lives. Their website provides information, resources, networking opportunities, and other tools for success. www.add.org
Centers for Disease Control and Prevention (CDC): Attention-Deficit/Hyperactivity Disorder (ADHD): www.cdc.gov/ncbddd/adhd/index.html
Center for Parent Information & Resources (CPIR): The CPIR is "the central hub of valuable information and products specifically designed for the network of Parent Centers serving families of children with disabilities." www.parentcenterhub.org.
Benjamin and Sarah Cheyette: The authors of this book regularly post in an ADHD blog on the *Psychology Today* website called "1-2-3 ADHD" at www.psychologytoday.com/us/blog/1-2-3-adhd. Sarah also has an informational website, SarahCheyette.com.

Children and Adults with Attention Deficit-Hyperactivity Disorder (CHADD): CHADD is a non-profit organization with chapters in many communities and over 12,000 members. Its mission is to improve the lives of people affected by ADHD using a set of core values. CHADD's Parent to Parent Program provides basic education on many facets of ADHD. www.chadd.org

Honestly ADHD: "A safe and supportive space dedicated to understanding and embracing life with ADHD." Provides "tips and strategies for everyday ADHD Life." honestlyadhd.com

National Organization for Learning Disabilities (NCLD): The NCLD, founded in 1977, aims to improve the lives of children and adults who have learning and attention disorders. It provides resources and advocates for equal rights for these individuals. www.ncld.org

Schwab Foundation for Learning—Internet Special Education Resources (ISER): ISER provides information, support, and hope for parents and educators helping kids with learning disabilities. Information about testing, treatments, programs, and more can be found on their website, http://www.iser.com/

Springboard Clinic: *May We Have Your Attention Please: A Springboard Clinic Workbook for Living—and Thriving—with Adult ADHD.* https://springboardclinic.com/resource/may-we-have-your-attention-please/

Understood.org: This nonprofit organization provides information and resources for ADHD and learning disabilities. https://www.understood.org/topics/school-supports

ADHD Coaches

ADHD Coaches Organization (ACO): The ACO is the worldwide professional membership organization for ADHD coaches. Their website provides information about ADHD coaches and helps clients select a coach. www.adhdcoaches.org

Coaching specifically for parents
>ADHD Essentials: Online parent coaching groups: https://www.adhdessentials.com/parentgroups
>Impact Parents—Helping Parents Help Kids: impactparents.com
>Sanity School: sanityschool.com

Edge Foundation: https://edgefoundation.org

Perler, Seth: Specializes in executive functioning coaching for students: https://sethperler.com

Podcasts
>"ADHD Essentials," Brendan Mahan: https://www.adhdessentials.com
>"Attention Talk Radio," Jeff Copper of DIG Coaching Practice: https://digcoaching.com/meet-jeff-copper
>"Taking Control," Terry Matlen: addconsults.com

Professional Association for ADHD Coaches (PAAC): PaacCoaches.org

Books

ADHD 2.0 by Dr. Edward Hallowell
ADHD: A Hunter in a Farmer's World by Thom Hartmann
ADHD & Me (picture book aimed at children, available on Amazon) by Dr. Sarah Cheyette and Dr. Benjamin Cheyette
ADHD & The Focused Mind (about using the athletic mindset to tackle ADHD challenges) by Dr. Sarah Cheyette and Dr. Benjamin Cheyette
Brain Surfing & 31 Other Awesome Qualities of ADHD by Laurie Dupar
Confessions of an ADDiva by Linda Roggli
Driven to Distraction by Dr. Edward Hallowell
How to Reach and Teach Children with ADD/ADHD: Practical Techniques, Strategies and Interventions by Sandra Rief
Late, Lost and Unprepared by Joyce Cooper Kahn and Laurie Dietzel
Let's Fix It: A Magic Kit for ADHD Adults by Linda Roggli
More Attention, Less Deficit: Success Strategies for Adults with ADHD by Ari Tuckman
Practical Ideas That Really Work for Students with ADHD by Kathleen McConnell and Gail Ryser

Taking Charge of ADHD by Dr. Russell Barkley
That Crumpled Paper Was Due Last Week: Helping Disorganized and Distracted Boys Succeed in School and in Life by Ana Homayoun
The ADHD Effect on Marriage by Melissa Orlov
The Couple's Guide to Thriving with ADHD by Melissa Orlov
The Essential Guide to Raising Complex Kids with ADHD, Anxiety and More by Elaine Taylor-Klaus
The Guide to ADHD Coaching: How to Find an ADHD Coach and What To Do When You Get One by Dr. Alan Graham
The Power of Full Engagement: Managing Energy, Not Time, Is the Key to High Performance and Personal Renewal by Jim Loehr and Tony Schwartz
365 Ways to Succeed with ADHD by Laurie Dupar
Twelve Principles for Raising a Child with ADHD by Dr. Russell Barkley
Understand Your Brain, Get More Done by Ari Tuckman
Understanding Girls With ADHD by Kathleen Nadeau, Ellen Littman, and Patricia Quinn
What Your ADHD Child Wishes You Knew by Dr. Sharon Saline
Winning with ADHD (a practical toolbook for coping with ADHD, aimed at teens, young adults) by Dr. Sarah Cheyette and Dr. Benjamin Cheyette

Electronic Management

Several websites list digital tools to reduce distractions. Some of the more effective tools are App Detox, Self-control, Focuswriter, WriteRoom, Anti-Social, StayFocusd, LeechBlock, Isolator, Freedom, and One Sec. For parents trying to manage their children's usage: MeetCircle, Qustodio, OurPact, Freedom.

Videogame Apps

EndeavorRx or EndeavorOTC: https://www.akiliinteractive.com/
Skylar's Run: https://thynk.com

Smartphone Apps

Mindfulness
  Buddhify: Buddhify.com
  Calm: Calm.com
  Headspace: Headspace.com
  Smiling Mind: smilingmind.com
Task management: Omnifocus (for Mac/ios) is an excellent system for managing tasks (https://www.omnigroup.com/omnifocus/). It will remind you to do things as you get closer to the building (for instance, when you pass the drugstore, it will remind you to pick up your prescriptions).
"To-do" lists
  Any.do
  ticktick.com
  todoist.com
Tracking time (spent or wasted)
  FocusBooster: Focusboosterapp.com
  Forest App: www.forestapp.cc/
  RescueTime: RescueTime.com

Educational Aids for Students

Camps and educational programs including boarding schools for ADHD kids and young adults ages 8 to 25: soarnc.org
Colleges
  Beacon College provides liberal arts degree programs for students with ADHD and learning disabilities (www.beaconcollege.edu).
  Landmark College in Vermont has a similar mission (www.landmark.edu).

Essay-writing: Templates for how to approach written language tasks can be helpful (such as how to write a persuasive essay or a creative story). Inspiration software is designed to improve organization and written composition skills. Inspiration 11/Mind Mapping and Graphic Organizers (inspiration-at.com).

Literacy technology
  Kurzweil software (www.kurzweiledu.com)
  https://learningally.org/

Math facts
  ABCya.com
  mathplayground.com

Note-taking
  Livescribe (https://us.livescribe.com/collections/smartpens) and other smart pen manufacturers
  SimpleNote: simplenote.com

Getting a 504 Plan or IEP

Consider asking your school about a 504 plan or an IEP. This is arranged through the school. Accommodations can be made such as extra time for tests, scheduling core classes in the morning, or sitting in areas with minimal distractions. Having a 504 plan or an IEP makes it much easier to get accommodations for standardized testing such as the SAT/ACT.

This type of evaluation is your legal right. To request the evaluation, you must write a brief note or letter stating that as the child's parents, you are concerned about areas in which he/she is struggling and how this may affect his/her learning at school, and in order to address those concerns, you request the psychoeducational evaluation. The school must respond within a specified amount of time (typically 60 days).

The following is a sample template that can be used when requesting a psychoeducational evaluation through the school:

[Date]
[Name of Principal]
[Name of School]
[Street Address]
[City, State, Zip]

Dear [Mr./Ms. Principal's Name],

Re: [Insert Your Child's Name Here]

I am hereby requesting that [Insert Name of County] School District conduct a complete and thorough Psychoeducational Assessment (to include intellectual, cognitive processing, and academic assessments) for my child. These are some of the areas about which I have concerns:

[Parents: choose all that apply, delete those that don't, feel free to add others not listed]

>   Reading
>   Math
>   Inability to do writing projects
>   Poor academic progress to date despite informal classroom accommodations
>   Behavioral problems in the classroom
>   Inability to pay attention
>   Cannot transition between activities
>   Forgets to bring papers, books, and homework home
>   Forgets to turn in homework
>   Very disorganized
>   Very anxious about going to school; doesn't like school
>   Poor social skills: does not have friends, or only has a few friends
>   Doesn't know how to appropriately interact with peers
>
>   Other areas: _____

I understand the school district has a limited time in which to complete these evaluations. Please accept this letter as my full consent to conduct the testing. I understand that I have the right to know the problem area(s) you have identified, the specific intervention(s) you plan to use to help my child, the person(s) responsible for implementing the plan, and a summary of the progress (or lack of progress) my child is making with the intervention once underway.

Thank you for your attention to this matter and for helping my child receive a free appropriate public education.

Sincerely,

[Parent's Name]
[Parent's Phone Number]
[Parent's Street Address]
[City, State, Zip]

APPENDIX 2

HII-5

Hyperactivity, Impulsivity, Inattention Symptom Rating Scale

Over the last <u>week</u>, how often have you been bothered by the following challenges?

	Not at all	Several days	More than half the days	Nearly every day
Fidgeting or difficulty sitting still	0	1	2	3
Interrupting other people or acting impulsively	0	1	2	3
Procrastinating on starting tasks	0	1	2	3
Starting but not finishing tasks	0	1	2	3
Mind wandering or forgetting what you were doing or saying	0	1	2	3

_____+_____+_____ +_____

= Total score: _____

If you checked off any challenges, how difficult have they made it for you to do your work, take care of things at home, or get along with other people?

Not difficult   Somewhat difficult   Very difficult   Extremely difficult
(managing well)   (debilitating)

Over the last week, I have taken ADHD medications (choose one):

- Every day
- On each day I needed them (but not 7 days/week)
- Intermittently (I forgot on some days when I should have taken them)
- Not at all

Note: The HII-5 is a rapid screening and symptom severity tracking tool. It was neither designed nor validated for establishing an ADHD diagnosis.

ABOUT *BRAIN & LIFE*® AND THE AMERICAN ACADEMY OF NEUROLOGY

The *Brain & Life* family of products includes a magazine, website, podcast, and book series. A print subscription to *Brain & Life*® (six issues a year) is available for free to anyone residing in the United States. Visit *BrainandLife.org* to subscribe or read stories on the latest information on treatments, managing neurologic conditions, and advice for keeping your brain as healthy as possible.

Brain & Life is an official publication of the American Academy of Neurology (AAN), the world's largest community of neurologists and neuroscience professionals and a leading voice in brain health. The neurologists at the AAN are the minds behind *Brain & Life*. A neurologist is a doctor who specializes in the diagnosis, care, and treatment of brain, spinal cord, and nervous system disease. That can include disorders like Alzheimer's disease, stroke, concussion, epilepsy, Parkinson's disease, multiple sclerosis, headache and migraine, and more. Learn more about the AAN's commitment to brain health for all at *AAN.com*.

INDEX

For the benefit of digital users, indexed terms that span two pages (e.g., 52–53) may, on occasion, appear on only one of those pages.

Tables and figures are indicated by an italic *t* and *f* following the page number.

absence seizures, 102–3
accommodations, defined, 223–25. *See also* school challenges and accommodations; work challenges and accommodations
ADD (attention-deficit disorder), 6, 31, 201, 223–25
ADD Coach Academy, 138
Adderall, 107, 115–16, 121*f*, 125, 126*t*, 127*t*
addiction
  dopamine and, 59
  fears of, 109
  high school years, 185–86
  mimicking or worsening ADHD, 98
  off-label medications, 130
  postnatal drug use, 67–68
  stimulants, 107, 120, 130

ADDitude magazine, 21
ADHD (attention-deficit/hyperactivity disorder), 6
  ADD versus, 6, 201
  balance when thinking about and describing aspects of, 219–20
  biological basis for, 11, 49–64
  care partners, 203–18
  in children versus in adults, 9–11
  common symptoms of, 4, 10–11, 32–33
  conditions that mimic or worsen, 36, 83–103
  consequences for everybody, 2–4, 203
  defined, 4, 223–25
  diagnosis for, 23–48
  downsides of not treating, 11–19

ADHD (attention-deficit/hyperactivity disorder) (*cont.*)
   famous people with, 20–21
   focused state versus unfocused state, 6–8, 8*f*
   lifespan perspective, 174–202
   misdiagnosis and overdiagnosis, 4
   oversimplified information and misinformation about, 2, 79
   presentations of, 6, 61, 117, 201–2, 236–39
   prevalence of, 9, 236–39
   procrastination, 154–65
   resources for, 243
   school challenges and accommodations, 44, 166–70, 180–81
   self-help resources, 170–73
   societal and environmental factors, 65–82
   treatments for, 104–35, 136–53
   upsides of, 7–8, 19–22, 219–22
   work challenges and accommodations, 11–12, 14, 20, 170, 188–90
ADHD Coach Training Center, 138
ADHDers, defined, 223–25
adrenaline (epinephrine), 58–59, 223–25
adults with ADHD, 188–93
   becoming parents, 191–93
   breastfeeding, 192–93
   children with ADHD versus, 9–11, 174–75, 177
   diagnosis for, 33–34, 35
   diagnostic criteria in, 201–2
   downsides of not treating ADHD, 13–19
   example questions asked on initial evaluation, 28
   gender gap, 179–80
   goal setting, 143
   heredity (genetics), 60
   history of diagnosis, 31, 32
   medication, 106–7, 108, 134–35
   negative consequences for inaction, 162–63
   organization therapy, 152
   pregnancy, 192–93
   prevalence rates, 9
   procrastination, 163
   relationship challenges, 189–91
   role in the family, 193–96
   sleep, 99
   survey instruments, 39
   therapeutic approaches in, 196–200
   work challenges and accommodations, 170, 189–90
   See also parents with ADHD; significant others/partners of adults with ADHD
affect, 52, 223–25
affective dysregulation, 33–34
affective reactivity/lability, 10–11, 223–25
agoraphobia, 223–25
alcohol and alcoholism
   addiction, 98
   alcoholism as comorbid condition, 80–81
   attentional difficulties, 36
   high school years, 185–86

middle school years, 184
prenatal exposure, 67
alleles, 223–25
Alzheimer disease, 97–98
ambivalence, 156–57
American Medical
 Association, 113–14
American Psychiatric Association,
 9, 113–14
Americans with Disabilities Act,
 167, 170
amphetamine-based stimulants,
 121*f*, 121, 125–26,
 126*t*, 127*t*
amygdala, 51, 55, 223–25
angular gyrus, 54, 223–25
anorexia nervosa, 187
anterior cingulate cortex, 223–25
antidepressants, 5, 86, 114–15,
 131, 197
anxiety and anxiety disorders
 anxiety, defined, 223–25
 care partners, 209–10
 CBT, 140
 cognitive behavioral therapy,
  137, 140
 as comorbid conditions, 80, 81–
  82, 84, 90, 134, 138
 feedback loop, 90–91, 91*f*
 generalized anxiety disorder, 9,
  80, 81, 84, 86–87, 90, 131,
  137, 231
 high school years, 186–87
 insomnia, 100
 invisible symptoms of
  ADHD, 212–13
 link to ADHD, 13
 mimicking or worsening
  ADHD, 4, 36, 90–92

norepinephrine, 59
off-label medications, 131
poor sleep and, 98–99, 100, 118
pregnancy and medication
 stoppage, 193
prevalence of generalized
 anxiety disorder, 9
signs of generalized anxiety
 disorder, 90
thinking/focus part and
 emotional part of brain,
 91*f*, 91
TMS, 172–73
women, 180
Aptensio, 121*f*, 122–23, 124*t*
Aristotle, 50
armodafinil, 121*f*, 130
arsenic, 70, 223–25
artificial colors, 70–71
artificial ingredients, 70–71
ASD (autism spectrum disorder)
 behavioral strategies, 95–96
 defined, 223–25
 differences between ADHD
  and, 94
 mimicking or worsening
  ADHD, 94–96
aspirin, 70–71
atomoxetine, 116, 128*f*, 128, 129–
 30, 131, 132
attention-deficit disorder (ADD),
 6, 31, 201, 223–25
attention-deficit/hyperactivity
 disorder. *See* ADHD
attention network (central
 executive network [CEN];
 task-positive network
 [TPN]), 52, 54–55, 57–
 59, 228–29

autism spectrum disorder.
    See ASD
avoidance, 44–45, 139–40, 149–
    50, 160–61
Azstarys, 121*f*, 124*t*, 125

basal ganglia, 28, 52, 58*f*, 225–26
BDNF (brain-derived
    neurotrophic factor), 152–
    53, 225–26
benzodiazepines, 120
bioenvironmental correlation,
    66–67, 225–26. *See also*
    biology of ADHD; societal
    and environmental factors
biology of ADHD, 11, 49–64
    bioenvironmental
        factors, 66–67
    biology, defined, 225–26
    brain chemistry, 55–60
    brain development, 175–78
    brain function, 54–55
    brain growth, 53–54
    brain structures and anatomy,
        50–52, 53–54, 60
    heredity (genetics), 60–63
    implications of for diagnosis
        and treatment, 63–64
biomarkers, 41, 225–26
bipolar disorder
    defined, 225–26
    heritability of, 60
    mimicking or worsening
        ADHD, 92
    stimulants, 108, 119
blood pressure
    clear medical
        guidelines, 104–5
    nonstimulants, 128, 130

    off-label medications, 131
    stimulants, 119–20
blood tests, 23, 38, 46, 113, 225–26
brain-derived neurotrophic factor
    (BDNF), 152–53, 225–26
brain function
    brain chemistry, 55–60
    differences in, 54–60
    poor sleep and, 98–99, 101
    procrastination and, 154–55
brain scans, 23, 38, 46, 47, 53–54,
    60, 225–26
Brain SPECT, 47
brainstem, 57–58, 58*f*, 59
brain structures and
        anatomy, 50–54
    brain circuits/networks, 50–
        51, 225–26
    brain growth and development,
        53–54, 175–77
    brain regions, 50–52
    diagnostic implications
        of, 53–54
    differences in people with and
        without ADHD, 51
    head circumference, 175
breastfeeding, 192–93
bupropion, 128*f*, 131
Buspar, 128*f*, 131
buspirone, 128*f*, 131

caffeine, 67–68, 114, 115, 117, 118
cannabis, 12, 36, 67–68, 80–81,
    98, 120
cardiology and cardiologists, 23–
    24, 119–20, 226–28
care partners, 203–18
    activities for connecting to the
        ADHDer, 217–18

ADHDer's invisible symptoms, 212–14
anger, 205
balance of partnership, 204
defined, 203–4, 226–28
educating yourself about ADHD, 210
fears, 205–6
feelings and emotions of, 205–9
getting help, 209–11
guilt, 206–7
making time for yourself, 218
not dismissing feelings, 210
positive focus, 211–12
shame, 206
sharing some of the burden, 210–11
supporting versus stepping back, 214–16
taking care of your own ADHD, 211
caudate, 52, 226–28
causal versus correlational evidence, 66, 226–28
CBT (cognitive behavioral therapy), 137, 139–42, 148, 226–28
CDC (U.S. Centers for Disease Control and Prevention), 108
celebrating successes, 140, 143–44, 160, 161f, 161
CEN (central executive network; attention network; task-positive network [TPN]), 52, 54–55, 57–59, 228–29
cerebral cortex, 52, 57–59, 58f, 226–28
cerebral palsy, 31, 226–28

child neurologists, 31, 226–28
child psychiatrists, 31, 226–28
children with ADHD
adults with ADHD versus, 9–11, 174–202
brain development, 175–78
brain growth, 53
brain wave testing, 41
diagnostic criteria in, 201–2
downsides of not treating ADHD, 13–19
educational psychologists and testing, 45–46
example questions asked on initial evaluation, 27–28
exercise, 153
free and appropriate public education, 44
gender gap, 178–79
goal setting, 134–35, 143
heredity, 60
history of diagnosis, 30–31
initial evaluation, 26–28, 29
learning disabilities, 43–46
neuropsychological testing, 43–44
organization therapy, 151–52
prevalence rates, 9
procrastination, 156–57, 159, 164–65
role in the family, 193–96
sleep, 99
survey instruments, 38–39
talk-based approaches, 141–42
testing for learning disabilities, 44
therapeutic approaches in, 196–200
See also parents of children with ADHD; school challenges and accommodations

clonidine, 116, 128*f*, 128, 129, 130, 132
coaching
 affordability, 138–39
 celebrating successes, 143–44
 children versus adults, 197
 choosing, 138–39
 coaches, defined, 223–25
 communication skills, 150–51
 to-do lists and reminders, 147
 exercise, 152–53
 goal setting, 142–43
 identifying your lies, 147
 interval training, 146
 resources regarding, 244–46
 rest and relaxation, 152
 sleep, 153
 therapy versus, 137–39
 time management, 145–46
cocaine, 67–68, 120
cognitive behavioral therapy (CBT), 137, 139–42, 148, 226–28
cognitive rigidity, 94–95
communication skills
 ADHD versus ASD, 95
 improving, 150–51
comorbid conditions, 80–82, 89, 119, 134, 138, 190–91
 anxiety, 90
 ASD, 94
 comorbid/comorbidity, defined, 226–28
 learning disabilities, 43
 masked symptoms, 81
 OCD, 92–93
computed tomography (CT), 50–51, 226–28
Concerta, 121*f*, 122–23, 124*t*

consistency index, 40
continuous performance tasks, 41–43
coping mechanisms, 98–99, 149–50, 191–92, 213–14
copper, 71
corpus callosum, 51, 52, 226–28
correlational versus causal evidence, 66, 226–28
Cotempla, 123, 124*t*
couples therapy, 151
"crazy busy" lives, 75–79
 historical changes to the simple act of getting to work, 75
 increase in ADHD diagnosis and, 78–79
 overscheduled and under-rested, 75
 superficial focus, 76
 switching tasks, 75–76
CT (computed tomography), 50–51, 226–28
cycle of failure, 226–28
cycle of success, 110, 144, 161*f*, 226–28

DAT (dopamine transporter) scans, 60, 228–29
Daytrana, 123, 124*t*
DBT (dialectical behavioral therapy), 141–42, 228–29
DEA (U.S. Drug Enforcement Agency), 130
default mode network (DMN), 51–52, 54–55, 176
dementia, 59, 96–98
depression, 86, 144, 191–92, 196
 antidepressants, 5, 86, 114–15, 131, 197

bipolar disorder, 92
care partners, 209–10
CBT, 140
  as comorbid condition, 80, 81, 89, 134, 138
  defined, 228–29
  dopamine and, 59
  high school years, 186–87
  insomnia, 100
  invisible symptoms of ADHD, 212–13
  major depressive disorder and episodes, 9, 29–30, 36, 62, 80, 81, 86–87
  mimicking or worsening ADHD, 4, 36, 84, 89, 90–92
  norepinephrine and, 59
  postpartum, 193
  symptoms and signs of, 89
  TMS, 172–73
  women, 180
developmental delay, 31, 228–29
Dexedrine, 121*f*, 125, 126*t*
dextroamphetamine, 121*f*, 125, 126, 126*t*
diabetes, 13, 104–5, 228–29
diagnosis for ADHD, 23–48
  children versus adults, 201–2
  compensating for symptoms, 35
  conditions that mimic ADHD, 36
  current criteria for, 32–38
  evolution of, 33–34
  finding the right professional, 23–26
  history of, 29–32
  hyperactivity and impulsivity-related symptoms, 33
  impact on multiple areas of life, 35
  implications of biology for, 63–64
  inattention-related symptoms, 32–33
  initial evaluation, 26–29
  meaningful impact on daily life, 36–38
  "no other reason," 36
  quantitative versus qualitative, 37, 239
  tests for, 38–48
  underdiagnosis in marginalized communities, 79
Diagnostic and Statistical Manual of Psychiatric Disorders (DSM-5)
  ADHD, 6, 9, 31, 32–34, 36, 37–38, 201, 202
  anxiety, 90
  ASD, 94
  defined, 228–29
  depression, 89
diagnostic mimicry and exacerbation, 36, 83–103
  addiction, 98
  ASD, 94–96
  dementia, 96–98
  diagnostic mimicry, defined, 228–29
  medical conditions, 101–3
  psychiatric conditions, 84–94
  sleep disorders and poor sleep, 98–101
dialectical behavioral therapy (DBT), 141–42, 228–29
dietary supplements, 71, 115, 133–34

"disappointing early," 150–51
dissociation, 228–29
distanced self-talk, 148
DMN (default mode network), 51–52, 54–55, 176
DMN interference model, 55, 228–29
dopamine, 57–58, 58f, 59, 115
  defined, 228–29
  nonstimulants, 116–17, 129
  off-label medications, 131
  stimulants, 116–17, 125
dopamine transporter (DAT) scans, 60, 228–29
dorsomedial prefrontal cortex, 54, 228–29
driving, 19, 35, 110, 165, 186, 189–90, 220
dyslexia, 43, 45, 46

educational psychologists and testing, 45–46, 137
EEG (electroencephalography), 41, 72, 102–3, 172–73, 228–29
electronic devices, 72–74, 98
  artificiality and passivity, 73
  FDA-approved devices and videogames, 73
  management aids, 246
  persistence, 73
  procrastination and, 155, 164–65
  recommended screen time, 73–74
  smartphone apps, 247
  speed of media presentation, 72
  type of device and usage, 72
  videogame apps, 246

elimination diets, 71
encephalitis lethargica (sleeping sickness), 30–31
EndeavorOTC, 171–72
EndeavorRx, 171–72
environmental factors. *See* societal and environmental factors
enzymes, 57, 115, 126
epidemiology
  correlational versus causal evidence, 66–67
  defined, 65–66, 228–29
epilepsy (seizure disorders), 31, 102, 228–29
epinephrine (adrenaline), 58–59, 223–25
Evekeo, 121f, 125, 126t
executive functioning, 53, 94–95, 141–42, 150, 172, 177–78, 180, 184, 197, 228–29
exercise, 12, 13, 85–86, 95–96, 146, 152–53, 218

family medicine, 25, 230
FAPE (free and appropriate public education), 44
FDA (U.S. Food and Drug Administration)
  brain wave testing, 41
  genetic testing, 113–14
  medications for adults versus for children, 10–11, 197
  medications for ASD versus for ADHD, 96
  off-label medications, 131
  pregnancy and medications, 192–93
  stimulants and nonstimulants, 115–16, 121, 128

technology-based treatments, 73, 171–73
FedEx Office and Print Services (Kinko's), 21
Feingold, Benjamin, 70
Feingold Diet, 70–71
504 plans, 44, 167, 168, 169–70, 215–16, 223–25, 248–50
Focalin, 115–16, 121*f*, 123*t*, 124–25, 124*t*
free and appropriate public education (FAPE), 44
Freud, Sigmund, 139
frontal lobe, 230

gender. *See* sex and gender
generalized anxiety disorder, 80, 81, 84, 86–87, 131, 137
   defined, 231
   prevalence of, 9
   symptoms and signs of, 90
general practice and practitioners, 25
genetics. *See* heredity
genetic testing, 38, 46–47, 61, 62, 63–64
   defined, 231
   to optimize choice of medication, 113–15
genome, 61–62
goal setting, 142–43
guanfacine, 116, 128*f*, 128, 129, 130, 132

Harvard Medical School, 32
heart disease, 13, 231–32
heavy metals, 70, 231–32
heredity (genetics), 60–63, 195
   chance and, 62–63
   complexity of, 61–62
   genes, defined, 231
   genetic testing, 38, 46–47, 61, 62, 113–15
   heritability, defined, 231–32
   heritability of ADHD, 60
   paleogenetics, 78–79, 236–39
   presentations of ADHD and, 61
heroin, 67
HII-5 symptom rating scale, 133, 251
hippocampus, 51–52, 54, 176, 231–32
historical development of ADHD diagnosis, 29–32
   ADD, 31
   adult ADHD, 31
   hyperkinetic impulse disorder, 30–31
   minimal brain dysfunction, 31
   moral disorder, 30, 31–32
   variation in classification, 29–30
Huntington chorea, 59
hyperactivity, 4, 6, 10–11
   anxiety, 90
   ASD, 95–96
   continuous performance task, 41
   defined, 231–32
   describing positively, 219
   distribution of symptoms in population, 37*f*, 37–38
   environmental factors, 65–66, 70–71
   family reaction, 194
   gender, 179
   heritability of ADHD, 61
   history of diagnosis, 30–31
   lifespan perspective, 201

hyperactivity (*cont.*)
  poor sleep and, 100
  presentations of ADHD, 61, 117, 201–2
  school challenges, 181, 182
  survey instruments, 39–40
  symptoms related to, 33
hyperfocus, 21–22, 147
hyperkinetic activity and hyperkinetic impulse disorder, 30–31, 70
hypomania, 92, 231–32

IDEA (Individuals with Disabilities Education Act), 44, 167–68
identical twins, 61, 62, 63
IEPs (individual education plans) and evaluations, 44, 45, 167–68, 199, 232–33, 248–50
impulsivity, 3, 6, 8, 10–11, 12, 13, 19, 22, 31, 83–84, 105, 106, 189–91
  ASD, 94–96
  bipolar disorder, 92
  defined, 232–33
  distribution of symptoms in population, 37*f*, 37–38
  driving, 186
  electronic devices, 73, 171, 190
  evaluation, 26–27, 28
  gender, 179
  heritability of ADHD, 61
  hyperkinetic impulse disorder, 30–31
  improving communication skills, 150–51
  lifespan perspective, 201
  medication, 86–87, 109–10, 129
  poor sleep and, 98–99, 153
  pregnancy, 193
  presentations of ADHD, 61, 201–2
  school challenges, 181, 182, 184, 185
  situation selection awareness, 148–49
  survey instruments, 39–40
  symptoms related to, 33
  THC, 67–68, 98
  upsides of, 19–20, 220–21
inattentiveness, 4, 6, 10–11, 12, 30, 31, 37–38, 190–91
  absence seizures, 102–3
  anxiety, 90
  continuous performance task, 41
  defined, 232–33
  depression, 36, 89
  distribution of symptoms in population, 37*f*, 37–38
  environmental factors, 65–66
  heritability of ADHD, 61
  high school years, 184–87
  improving communication skills, 150
  lifespan perspective, 201
  medication, 110, 117
  presentations of ADHD, 61, 117, 201–2
  survey instruments, 39–40
  symptoms related to, 32–33
individual education plans (IEPs) and evaluations, 44, 45, 167–68, 199, 232–33, 248–50

Individuals with Disabilities Education Act (IDEA), 44, 167–68
insomnia, 100, 101, 118, 232–33. *See also* sleep disorders and poor sleep
internal medicine and internists, 25, 232–33
interval training, 146
Intuniv, 116, 128*f*, 128
in utero
  brain development, 63, 175–76
  defined, 232–33
  drug exposure, 67
  mothers with ADHD, 192–93
  stress exposure, 68–69
iron, 71, 133–34

JetBlue Airlines, 21
Jornay, 121*f*, 123–24, 124*t*

Kapvay, 116, 128
Kinko's (FedEx Office and Print Services), 21

LCSWs (licensed clinical social workers), 137
lead exposure, 70
learning disabilities, 43–44, 45, 46, 94–95, 167–68
LEPs (licensed educational psychologists), 137
limbic system, 51–52, 58*f*, 58–59, 176, 233
lisdexamfetamine, 115–16
L-methylfolate, 115
LMFTs (licensed marriage and family therapists), 137
loci, 61–62, 233

LPCCs (licensed professional clinical counselors), 137

magnetic resonance imaging (MRI), 50–51, 233–34
major depressive disorder and episodes, 29–30, 81
  as comorbid condition, 80
  defined, 233–34
  genetics, 62
  inattentiveness, 36
  medication stops working, 86–87
  prevalence of episodes, 9
  See also depression
mania
  bipolar disorder, 92
  defined, 233–34
  hypomania, 92, 231–32
marginalized communities, 79
Mark, Gloria, 76
medication, 104–35
  addiction, 109
  antidepressants, 131, 197
  ASD versus ADHD, 95–96
  brand-name versus generic, 126–28
  children versus adults, 197–98
  choosing a medication, 112–13
  deciding whether to use, 104–8, 110–12
  dietary supplements, 133–34
  dosing, 132–33
  downsides of not treating ADHD, 105–6
  expectations regarding, 109–10
  frequency of doctor's visits for management of, 133
  genetic testing, 113–15

medication (*cont.*)
   lack of clear medical guidelines, 104–5, 112
   lack of objectivity, 106–7
   limitations of, 134–35
   nonstimulants, 115–17, 128–30
   off-label medications, 130–31
   overprescription, 4, 108
   parental fears regarding, 108–9
   pregnancy and breastfeeding, 192–93
   risk for anorexia nervosa, 187
   stigma and misconceptions, 107
   stimulants, 115–26
   tolerance for, 133
   usage rates, 108
   when medication stops working, 86–87
   when other strategies have failed, 110
melancholia, 29–30
mental status exams, 26–27
mercury, 70
Metadate, 123*t*
methamphetamine, 67–68
Methylin, 123*t*
methylphenidate-based stimulants, 121*f*, 121, 122–25, 123*t*, 124*t*
mimicking conditions. *See* diagnostic mimicry and exacerbation
mindfulness, 141, 148
minimal brain dysfunction, 31
modafinil, 121*f*, 130
monoamines, 57, 233–34
mood disorders, 36, 80, 82. *See also* depression; major depressive disorder and episodes
MRI (magnetic resonance imaging), 50–51, 233–34
Mydayis, 121*f*, 126, 127*t*
myelination, 175–76, 233–34

National Institutes of Health (NIH), 32, 53
NEBA (neuropsychiatric EEG-based assessment aid) system, 41, 234–36
Neeleman, David, 21
negativity bias, 144, 211–12, 234–36
neurodevelopmental disorders, 4, 70, 234–36
neurons, 55–57, 56*f*, 152–53, 175–76, 234–36
neuropsychiatric conditions, 6, 47, 59, 62–63, 68–69, 113–14
neuropsychiatric EEG-based assessment aid (NEBA) system, 41, 234–36
neuropsychiatry and neuropsychiatrists, 45–46, 234–36
neuropsychological testing, 41–43, 45–46, 234–36
neurotoxins, 70
neurotransmitter receptors, 56*f*, 56–57, 234–36
neurotransmitters, 55–59, 56*f*
   defined, 234–36
   nonstimulants, 117, 129
   stimulants, 115, 116
nicotine, 66–68, 131
NIH (National Institutes of Health), 32, 53

nonstimulants
  dosing, 132
  function of, 129
  relationships between, 128*f*
  side effects of, 128
  stimulants versus, 129–30
nootropics, 134
norepinephrine (noradrenaline), 57, 58*f*, 58–59, 115, 125
  antidepressants, 131
  defined, 234–36
  nonstimulants, 58–59, 129
  off-label medications, 131
  stimulants, 58–59
NPs (nurse practitioners), 24, 25–26
nucleus accumbens, 51, 234–36
Nuvigil, 121*f*, 130

obstructive sleep apnea, 101–2, 130
OCD (obsessive–compulsive disorder), 92–93, 172–73, 236
off-label medications, 121*f*, 130–31
omega-3 fatty acids, 71, 133–34
Onyda, 116, 128, 130
Orfalea, Paul, 21
organization therapy, 151–52

paleogenetics, 78–79, 236–39
panic disorders and attacks, 59, 87–88, 114, 137, 149, 236–39
parent–child interaction therapy, 141–42, 236–39
parent management training, 141–42, 236–39

parents of children with ADHD, 3
  bioenvironmental factors, 66–67
  child's role in the family, 194–95
  coaching versus therapy, 138
  "crazy busy" lives, 75
  feelings and emotions of, 204, 206–7
  heritability of ADHD, 60, 195, 216
  medication, 106–7, 108–9, 112
  organization therapy, 151–52
  parent–child interaction therapy, 141–42, 236–39
  parent management training, 141–42, 236–39
  procrastination, 156–57
  supporting versus stepping back, 29, 215
  talk-based approaches, 141–42
  See also children with ADHD; school challenges and accommodations
parents with ADHD, 9–10, 191–93, 195
  adult children of older parents with ADHD, 3–4
  family conflict, 69–70
  medication, 198
  pregnancy and breastfeeding, 192–93
  stress exposure, 69
parietal lobe, 236–39
Parkinson's disease, 59
partners of adults with ADHD. *See* care partners; significant others/partners of adults with ADHD

pathological processes and behaviors, 7–8, 236–39
pediatrics and pediatricians, 25, 31, 178–79, 199, 236–39
penetrance, 62, 236–39
PET (positron emission tomography), 54, 236–39
physicians, 10–11, 24–26, 30, 31, 47, 81
play therapy, 141–42, 236–39
PMHNPs (psychiatric and mental health nurse practitioners), 25–26, 236–39
Pomodoro method and apps, 146, 171
positron emission tomography (PET), 54, 236–39
posterior cingulate cortex (precuneus), 54, 236–39
post-traumatic stress disorder (PTSD), 137, 236–39
poverty, 66–67, 69–70, 106
prefrontal cortex, 129, 177–78, 236–39
pregnancy
  ADHD in pregnant mothers, 192–93
  causal versus correlational evidence, 66–67
  child brain development during, 175–76
  prenatal exposure to drugs, 67
  prenatal exposure to stress, 68–69
presentations of ADHD, 6, 61, 117, 201–2, 236–39
prevalence of ADHD, 9, 236–39
procrastination, 5, 8, 33, 77, 87–88, 107, 109, 111, 144, 149–50, 154–65, 169
  brain function, 154–55
  breaking tasks down into smaller chunks, 160, 161*f*
  depression, 89
  electronic distractions, 164–65
  getting help with personal blocks, 159
  identifying ambivalence, 156–57
  imposing negative consequences for inaction, 162–64
  improving time management, 145–46
  procrastivity, 162
  reasons behind, 154–56
  scheduling dreaded tasks early, 160–62
  school challenges, 184–85
  self-deceptions, 147
  skills for management of, 159–65
  starting with smallest bit, 159, 160*f*
  understanding the ADHDer's viewpoint, 157–59
procrastivity, 162
Provigil, 121*f*, 130
psychiatric and mental health nurse practitioners (PMHNPs), 25–26, 236–39
psychiatry and psychiatrists, 5, 24, 25, 31, 32, 137, 236–39
psychoactive drugs, 67–68
psychoanalysis, 139, 236–39
psychological stress, 68–70, 88
  during childhood and adolescence, 69–70
  during infancy, 69
  prenatal exposure, 68–69

psychology and psychologists, 2, 24–25, 45–46, 137, 180–81, 236–39
psychosis, 59, 93–94, 193, 236–39
PTSD (post-traumatic stress disorder), 137, 236–39
putamen, 52, 236–39

Qelbree, 116, 128f, 128
quantitative versus qualitative diagnosis, 37, 239
QuilliChew, 123, 124t
Quillivant, 123, 124t

recall bias, 40
Rehabilitation Act of 1973, 44, 167
resources for ADHD, 243
　books, 245
　coaches, 244–46
　educational aids for students, 247–48
　electronic management aids, 246
　504 plans and IEPs, 248–50
　smartphone apps, 247
　videogame apps, 246
　websites, 243–44
rest and relaxation, 152. *See also* sleep disorders and poor sleep
retrospective studies, 66, 239
Ritalin, 115–16, 121f, 122–23, 124–26, 124t

salience network (SN), 51, 55, 240–41
schizophrenia
　defined, 240
　dopamine and, 59
　heritability of, 60, 62
　mimicking or worsening ADHD, 93–94
　stimulants, 108, 119
school challenges and accommodations, 44, 166–70, 180–81
　college, 169, 187–88
　elementary school, 182
　504 plans, 44, 167, 168, 169–70, 215–16, 223–25, 248–50
　high school, 184–87
　IEPs and evaluations, 44, 45, 167–68, 199, 232–33, 248–50
　middle school, 183–84
　preschool, 181–82
　pros and cons of, 168–69
seizure disorders (epilepsy), 31, 102, 228–29
self-deceptions, 147
self-help resources, 170–73
　electronic management aids, 171, 246
　technology-based treatments, 171–73, 246
self-medication, 67–68, 185–86
sex and gender
　biological factors, 178–80
　defined, 178
　gender biases, 9
　presentations of ADHD and, 61
　prevalence of ADHD, 9
sexually transmitted diseases (STDs), 13, 105, 190–91, 240
significant others/partners of adults with ADHD
　assessment of ADHDer and, 201
　couples therapy, 151

significant others/partners of adults with ADHD (*cont.*)
  feelings and emotions of, 3, 17–18, 204, 205
  organization therapy, 151–52
  relationship challenges, 190–91
  supporting versus stepping back, 29
  See also care partners
single photon emission computed tomography (SPECT), 54, 240
situation selection awareness, 148–50
Skylar's Run, 171–72
sleep apnea, 36, 101–2, 130
sleep disorders and poor sleep
  brain function, 98–99, 101
  as comorbid conditions, 82
  getting sufficient sleep, 153
  insomnia, 100, 101, 118, 232–33
  mimicking or worsening ADHD, 98–101
  prevalence of, 99
  recommended hours of sleep, 99–100
  side effects of stimulants, 118
  sleep apnea, 36, 101–2, 130
  "sleeping in," 100
sleeping sickness (encephalitis lethargica), 30–31
smartphone apps, 247. *See also* electronic devices
SN (salience network), 51, 55, 240–41
societal and environmental factors, 65–82
  artificial colors and ingredients, 70–71
  bioenvironmental factors, 66–67
  correlational versus causal evidence, 66
  "crazy busy" lives, 75–79
  dietary supplements, 71
  drug use, 67–68
  electronic distractions/diversions, 72–74
  marginalized communities, 79
  other mental health challenges, 80–82
  psychological stress, 68–70
  sugar, 70
  toxins, 70
SPECT (single photon emission computed tomography), 54, 240
STDs (sexually transmitted diseases), 13, 105, 190–91, 240
stimulants
  amphetamine-based, 121*f*, 121, 125–26, 126*t*, 127*t*
  dosing, 132
  function of, 116
  immediate-release versus longer-acting, 121*f*, 121–22, 123*t*, 124*t*, 126*t*, 127*t*
  methylphenidate-based, 121*f*, 121, 122–25, 123*t*, 124*t*
  most common, 115–16
  nonstimulants versus, 116–17, 129–30
  relationships between, 121*f*
  side effects of, 118–21
  stopping, 117
  types of, 121–26
  upsides of, 115–16

usage rates, 115–16
Strattera, 116, 128
substance use and abuse, 13, 67–68, 98, 106, 110
   addiction, 98, 120
   as comorbid condition, 80, 81, 98
   high school years, 185–86
   mimicking or worsening ADHD, 36
   postnatal, 67–68
   prenatal exposure, 67
sugar, 70
synapses, 55–57, 56*f*, 116, 129, 175–76, 240

talk-based approaches, 135, 136–53
   affordability, 138–39
   celebrating successes, 143–44
   children versus adults, 197
   coaching versus therapy, 137–39
   communication skills, 150–51
   couples therapy, 151
   distanced self-talk, 148
   to-do lists and reminders, 147
   exercise, 152–53
   goal setting, 142–43
   identifying your lies, 147
   interval training, 146
   licensed professionals, 137
   mindfulness, 148
   organization therapy, 151–52
   rest and relaxation, 152
   situation selection awareness, 148–50
   sleep, 153
   time management, 145–46
   types of, 139–42
   visualization, 145
task-positive network (TPN; central executive network [CEN]; attention network), 52, 54–55, 57–59, 228–29
technology-based treatments, 73, 171–73
   TMS, 172–73
   TNS, 172
   videogame systems and apps, 171–72, 246
Ted Lasso (TV show), 220
temporal cortex, 52, 240–41
THC, 67–68, 98
therapists, 1
   coaching versus therapy, 137–39
   defined, 240–41
   tips for therapy, 142–53
TMS (transcranial magnetic stimulation), 172–73, 240–41
TNS (trigeminal nerve stimulation), 172, 240–41
to-do lists and reminders, 18, 38, 77–78, 90, 147, 160, 171
tolerance, 133, 197–98, 240–41
toxins, 70
TPN (task-positive network; attention network; central executive network [CEN]), 52, 54–55, 57–59, 228–29
transcranial magnetic stimulation (TMS), 172–73, 240–41
treatments for ADHD
   children versus adults, 10–11, 196–200

treatments for ADHD (*cont.*)
  downsides of not treating ADHD, 11–12, 13–19, 105–6
  implications of biology for, 63–64
  medication, 104–35
  self-help resources, 170–73
  talk-based approaches, 135, 136–53
trigeminal nerve stimulation (TNS), 172, 240–41
triple network model, 55, 240–41

upsides of ADHD, 7–8, 19–22, 219–22
  big-picture thinking, 220
  creative thinking, 221–22
  curiosity, 220
  energy, 219–20
  reaction times, 220–21
  results-oriented activities, 221
  willingness to take risks, 221
urologists, 23–24
U.S. Centers for Disease Control and Prevention (CDC), 108
U.S. Department of Education, 44, 167
U.S. Drug Enforcement Agency (DEA), 130

U.S. Food and Drug Administration. *See* FDA

variants in the genome, 61–62, 78–79, 241–42
vicious cycles, 16, 19, 66–67, 90–91, 91*f*, 98, 153, 184–85, 241–42
videogame systems and apps, 72, 98, 171–72, 246
viloxazine, 116, 128*f*, 128, 129, 132
virtuous cycles, 6–7, 144, 161*f*, 241–42
visualization, 145, 162–63
vitamin D, 133–34
Vyvanse, 115–16, 121*f*, 126, 127*t*

website blockers, 171
Wellbutrin, 128*f*, 131
Whitman, Walt, 220
work challenges and accommodations, 11–12, 14, 20, 170, 188–90

Xelstrym, 127*t*

Zenzedi, 121*f*, 126*t*
zinc, 71, 133–34
zombification, 22, 198